T0295345

FETAL ALCOHOL SYNDROME

RECOGNITION, DIFFERENTIAL DIAGNOSIS AND LONG-TERM EFFECTS

PEDIATRICS – LABORATORY AND CLINICAL RESEARCH

Additional books and e-books in this series can be found
on Nova's website under the Series tab.

FETAL ALCOHOL SYNDROME

RECOGNITION, DIFFERENTIAL DIAGNOSIS AND LONG-TERM EFFECTS

DOUG KNIGHT
EDITOR

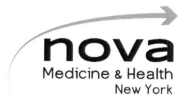

nova
Medicine & Health
New York

Copyright © 2018 by Nova Science Publishers, Inc.

All rights reserved. No part of this book may be reproduced, stored in a retrieval system or transmitted in any form or by any means: electronic, electrostatic, magnetic, tape, mechanical photocopying, recording or otherwise without the written permission of the Publisher.

We have partnered with Copyright Clearance Center to make it easy for you to obtain permissions to reuse content from this publication. Simply navigate to this publication's page on Nova's website and locate the "Get Permission" button below the title description. This button is linked directly to the title's permission page on copyright.com. Alternatively, you can visit copyright.com and search by title, ISBN, or ISSN.

For further questions about using the service on copyright.com, please contact:
Copyright Clearance Center
Phone: +1-(978) 750-8400   Fax: +1-(978) 750-4470   E-mail: info@copyright.com.

NOTICE TO THE READER

The Publisher has taken reasonable care in the preparation of this book, but makes no expressed or implied warranty of any kind and assumes no responsibility for any errors or omissions. No liability is assumed for incidental or consequential damages in connection with or arising out of information contained in this book. The Publisher shall not be liable for any special, consequential, or exemplary damages resulting, in whole or in part, from the readers' use of, or reliance upon, this material. Any parts of this book based on government reports are so indicated and copyright is claimed for those parts to the extent applicable to compilations of such works.

Independent verification should be sought for any data, advice or recommendations contained in this book. In addition, no responsibility is assumed by the publisher for any injury and/or damage to persons or property arising from any methods, products, instructions, ideas or otherwise contained in this publication.

This publication is designed to provide accurate and authoritative information with regard to the subject matter covered herein. It is sold with the clear understanding that the Publisher is not engaged in rendering legal or any other professional services. If legal or any other expert assistance is required, the services of a competent person should be sought. FROM A DECLARATION OF PARTICIPANTS JOINTLY ADOPTED BY A COMMITTEE OF THE AMERICAN BAR ASSOCIATION AND A COMMITTEE OF PUBLISHERS.

Additional color graphics may be available in the e-book version of this book.

Library of Congress Cataloging-in-Publication Data

Library of Congress Control Number: 2018960054
ISBN: 978-1-53614-602-8

Published by Nova Science Publishers, Inc. † New York

CONTENTS

PREFACE

Alcohol has long been a well renowned and leading teratogen that inflicts a myriad of adverse effects on the offspring exposed during pregnancy in alcoholic mothers, ranging from mild to severe malformed features. Fetal Alcohol Syndrome: Recognition, Differential Diagnosis and Long-Term Effects opens with a presentation on the diagnostic criteria for identifying and distinguishing these various alcohol-related disorders and their respective characteristic features.

There are considerable problems in diagnosing fetal alcohol spectrum disorders and evidence of more than minimal exposure to ethanol during pregnancy is an important criterion. Information on the mother's alcohol consumption during pregnancy may not be available or may be inaccurate. Furthermore, approximately half of children affected by may not exhibit signs until they are preschool or school-age. Thus, the authors assess emerging enduring markers of prenatal alcohol exposure.

The following chapter summarizes data from investigations of the effects of alcohol on neuron-microglia interactions based on recent findings which demonstrate that alcohol causes loss of both neurons and microglia in the developing brain. Structural and functional characteristics of neuron-microglia interactions are presented, as well as the effects of alcohol on various cytokines which play roles in the mechanisms of those interactions.

The various long-term effects of drinking during pregnancy on the immune and the neuroimmune systems of the developing fetus, baby and child are also discussed. The results suggest that fetal alcohol exposure induces long-term defects in the immunity and susceptibility to various infections.

Chapter 1 - Alcohol had long been a well renowned and leading teratogen that inflicts a myriad of consequences on the offspring exposed during pregnancy in alcoholic mothers, with assaults ranging from mild to severe malformed characteristics features. Reporters had described these different but related teratological features by different terminologies such as: Fetal Alcohol Syndrome (FAS), Fetal Alcohol Effect (FAE), Alcohol Related Birth Defects (ARBD), Fetal Alcohol Spectrum Disorder (FASD), Alcohol Related Neuro-developmental Disorder (ARND) and Partial Fetal Alcohol Syndrome (PFAS). However, critical observations had shown that there are no distinct diagnostic criteria to identify and distinguish these terminologies and FAS with their respective characteristic features. Hence, this chapter offers to present a clear and acceptable identity for FAS.

Chapter 2 - Fetal Alcohol Spectrum Disorders (FASD) is the term used to describe neurobehavioural disorders associated with prenatal alcohol exposure ranging from the most severe Fetal alcohol syndrome (FAS) with facial dysmorphology, through partial Fetal alcohol syndrome (pFAS) to alcohol-related birth defects (ARBD). Many of the cognitive impairments associated with FASD are similar to those seen in Attention Deficit Hyperactivity Disorder (ADHD), Autistic Spectrum Disorders and other such conditions. There are considerable problems in diagnosing FASD and evidence of more than minimal exposure to ethanol during pregnancy is an important criterion. Information on the mother's alcohol consumption during pregnancy may not be available, or may be inaccurate. Furthermore, approximately half of children affected by FASD may not exhibit signs of CNS dysfunction until they are preschool or school-age when the child and the mother may have become separated.

Early accurate differential diagnosis would enable the most effective treatments to be used. Ideally biomarkers would be identified which would enable confirmation of prenatal alcohol exposure. The use of meconium as an accessible fetal source of fatty acid ethyl esters (FAEEs), ethyl glucuronide (EtG) and ethyl sulfate (EtS) is frequently considered, but this is only applicable for the first few days of the neonate's life. The use of neonatal blood phosphatidylethanol (PEth) has also been discussed, but again the longevity of this biomarker is short. More recently results from animal studies of neonatal plasma microRNA biomarkers and changes to histone modifications have provided new opportunities, and DNA methylation has been suggested as a potential biomarker. The authors' own work suggests that prenatal alcohol exposure may induce long-lived changes in brain derived neurotrophic factor (BDNF) and brain aminopeptidase activity which may be reflected in changes in plasma or urine.

In the light of the evidence that many fetuses are exposed to alcohol but do not exhibit any degree of FASD, this review will assess the evidence of reliability of emerging enduring markers of prenatal alcohol exposure and explore whether they correlate only with prenatal alcohol exposure or also with FASD.

Chapter 3 - Fetal alcohol spectrum disorder (FASD) is a result of maternal consumption of alcohol during pregnancy. This chapter summarizes data from investigations of the effects of alcohol on neuron-microglia interactions. It is based on recent findings in models of FASD which demonstrate that alcohol causes loss of both neurons and microglia in the developing brain. The chapter presents structural and functional characteristics of neuron-microglia interactions as well as the effects of alcohol on various cytokines which play roles in the mechanisms of those interactions. The consequences of glial nitric oxide synthase activity in the apoptotic effects of ethanol on developing neurons are also illustrated. The key factors regulated by the microglia-specific signal transducer and activator of transcription 3 in neuron–microglia interactions are analyzed. Overall, the chapter summarizes the long-term effects of fetal alcohol exposure on neuronal plasticity.

Chapter 4 - Limited human studies have been conducted on the immune status of children with fetal alcohol spectrum disorder (FASD). The present review is aimed to fill up these gaps in knowledge. The chapter discusses various long-term effects of drinking during pregnancy on the immune and the neuroimmune systems of the developing fetus, baby and child. The results suggest that fetal alcohol exposure (FAE) induces long-term defects in the immunity and susceptibility to various infections. Mechanisms of impaired immune proliferation and function in FASD are a subject of the review. Chronic alcohol exposure in utero interferes with the normal T-cell and B-cell development of the fetus, which may increase the risk of infections during childhood and adult development. Influenza virus infection as well as increased risk for severe and fetal respiratory infections are illustrated in the long-term effects of FAE. Recognition of neuroimmunological dysfunctions due to developmental ethanol exposure and their lasting harmful effects in the early infancy and in the adulthood are also discussed in this chapter.

In: Fetal Alcohol Syndrome
Editor: Doug Knight

ISBN: 978-1-53614-602-8
© 2018 Nova Science Publishers, Inc.

Chapter 1

FETAL ALCOHOL SYNDROME: ITS DISTINGUISHING CHARACTERISTIC FEATURES

Samuel Sunday Adebisi, PhD
Department of Human Anatomy,
Ahmadu Bello University, Zaria, Nigeria

ABSTRACT

Alcohol had long been a well renowned and leading teratogen that inflicts a myriad of consequences on the offspring exposed during pregnancy in alcoholic mothers, with assaults ranging from mild to severe malformed characteristics features. Reporters had described these different but related teratological features by different terminologies such as: Fetal Alcohol Syndrome (FAS), Fetal Alcohol Effect (FAE), Alcohol Related Birth Defects (ARBD), Fetal Alcohol Spectrum Disorder (FASD), Alcohol Related Neuro-developmental Disorder (ARND) and Partial Fetal Alcohol Syndrome (PFAS). However, critical observations had shown that there are no distinct diagnostic criteria to identify and distinguish these terminologies and FAS with their respective characteristic features. Hence, this chapter offers to present a clear and acceptable identity for FAS.

INTRODUCTION

Fetal alcohol syndrome (FAS) could be aptly described as the manifestation of some salient physical and functional features of congenital anomalies in individuals that is due to their prenatal exposure to alcohol (Adebisi, 2002). Although FAS is a developmental enigma that had rather been with us for long but unnoticed, the first report on FAS was published by Lemoine and colleagues in 1968 in a study on 127 children of alcoholic mothers. But even so, FAS remained an unpopular subject until Jones and colleagues' publication in Lancet in 1973 on eight children born to chronic alcoholic mothers; this subsequently triggered wide researches and reports (Mednet, 2010). Alcohol had since then been recognized as a foremost but preventable teratogen capable of causing birth defects on the fetus likely to be exposed (Mednet, 2010).

SOURCE AND METABOLISM OF ETHANOL

Naturally, ethanol – the main toxic form of alcohol can be formed when fermentation is started in sugar containing plants by yeast (Brent, 1973):

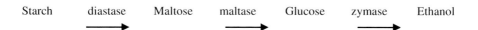

Starch   diastase   Maltose   maltase   Glucose   zymase   Ethanol

Ethanol is the mostly used and ingested form of the alcohol family. Its absorption commences even from the oral cavity and throughout the digestive tract. Metabolism and detoxification occur in the liver thus:

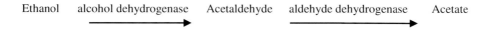

Ethanol   alcohol dehydrogenase   Acetaldehyde   aldehyde dehydrogenase   Acetate

Acetaldehyde as the main metabolite had been noted to be responsible for the morpho-toxicity of ethanol. Unlike in the mother's liver, alcohol cum acetaldehyde accumulates in the fetus since the developing fetal liver yet lacks the detoxifying enzymes which as at this time is not yet expressed (Sreenathan, 1982; Di Bartolo et al., 1987).

ALCOHOL AND PREGNANCY

There had been no adequate documentation of the maternal history of alcohol consumption during pregnancy, that is, the amount and timing of drinking during pregnancy. Problem drinkers are not easily identified just by their appearance or socioeconomic status. Binge drinking, that is, four or more drinks in one sitting is more problematic than consumption of the same amount of alcohol spread out over time, for instance, that is, one drink per day for four days. Alcohol ingested during pregnancy is rapidly transported via placental blood flow from mother to fetus and is known to cause abortion and birth defects. Within two hours of maternal ingestion, fetal alcohol blood levels are similar to maternal alcohol blood levels. Interestingly, alcohol could potentiate its toxicity on the fetal tissues throughout the gestational period as had been observed in the followings: first trimester pregnancy alcohol ingestion is linked to the characteristic facial abnormalities as well as a reduction of intrauterine growth rate. Alcohol consumption during the second trimester also contributes to lower IQ, growth retardation in length and birth weight, as well as cognitive deficits of reading and spelling. Third trimester alcohol consumption amplifies retardation in birth length and ultimate adult height potential. In this respect, total abstinence from alcohol for women planning pregnancy was recommended in the United States at the time of conception and throughout the entire pregnancy since no safe period or level of prenatal alcohol consumption has been documented (Bertrand et al., 2004). Although, it was observed that some children sustain no obvious side effects of maternal alcohol consumption during pregnancy, which perhaps could probably be attributed to differences in individual alcohol tolerance for instance, and this had been associated with their genetic factors (Poskitt, 1984; Di Bartolo and Carlos, 1987).

ALCOHOL BIRTH DEFECTS

Shortly following the earliest day of recognition of birth defects associated with alcohol use at pregnancy, different terminologies were, used to describe these anomalies. These include the followings:

Alcohol Related Birth Defects (ARBD)

This apparently appears as the germinal identity for these myriad of scourge. This term was, really meant to encompass all the observable ethanol associated congenital menace. It was, formerly known as Possible Fetal Alcohol Effect (PFAE). ARBD was, presented as a list of congenital anomalies that are linked to maternal alcohol use but have no specified key features (Committee, 1995). PFAE and ARBD however, have fallen out of favor because even the listed anomalies are not necessarily specific to maternal alcohol consumption and are not criteria for diagnosis of any of the fetal alcohol defects (Streissguth, 1997). More so, the Canadian guidelines recommend that ARBD should not be used as an umbrella term or diagnosis.

Fetal Alcohol Effects (FAE)

This was an earlier term describing alcohol-related neuro-developmental disorders and alcohol-related birth defects (FASD, 2015). It was initially used in research studies in humans and animals in whom teratogenic effects were seen after confirmed prenatal alcohol exposure (or unknown exposure for humans), but without obvious physical anomalies. Smith (1981) described FAE as an "extremely important concept" to highlight the debilitating effects of brain damage, regardless of the growth or facial features. However, this term had also now fallen out of favor particularly with clinicians because it was often given a picture of a less severe disability than FAS, when in fact its effects can be just as serious in the affected subjects (Clarren and Smith, 1978; Aase et al., 1995).

Alcohol-Related Neuro-Developmental Disorder (ARND)

Alcohol-related neuro-developmental disorder (ARND) also known as static encephalopathy was initially suggested by the Institute of Medicine to replace the term FAE and focus on central nervous system damage, rather than growth deficiency or FAS facial features defects. ARND may be gaining acceptance over the terms FAE and ARBD to describe FASD conditions with central nervous system abnormalities or behavioral or cognitive abnormalities or both due to prenatal alcohol exposure without regard to growth deficiency or FAS facial features defects (Streissguth 1997; Malbin, 2002). However, the following criteria must be fully met for a diagnosis of ARND or static encephalopathy according to the 'Ten brain domain' or the '4-Digit Diagnostic Code' which is the standardized or harmonized diagnostic criteria developed by the Institute of Health, the US Academy of Science and the Centre for Disease Control and Canadian guidelines for measuring CNS damage.

The criteria include:

- Growth deficiency: Growth or height may range from normal to minimally deficient
- FAS facial features: Minimal or no FAS facial features present
- Central nervous system damage: Clinically significant structural, neurological or functional impairment in three or more of the Ten Brain Domains
- Confirmed prenatal alcohol exposure.
  (Streissguth, 1997; Chudley et al., 2005; Committee, 2016; Astley, 2004; Clinical Growth Archived, 2010; FAS facial features Archived, 2007; Lang, 2006).

Fetal Alcohol Spectrum Disorders

(FASDs) refers to group of conditions that can occur in a person whose mother drank alcohol during pregnancy, but a clear working knowledge of the key features could be helpful in understanding FASDs. Problems may include an abnormal appearance, short height, low body weight, small head size, poor coordination, low intelligence, behavior problems, and problems with hearing or seeing. Central nervous system (CNS) damage is the primary key feature of any FASD diagnosis. Those affected are more likely to have trouble in school, legal problems, participate in high-risk behaviors, and have trouble with alcohol or other drugs. In terms of FASDs, growth deficiency is defined as significantly below average height, weight or both due to prenatal alcohol exposure, and can be assessed at any point in the lifespan of sufferers. More than 400 problems, however, can occur with FASDs (FASD, 2015; Committee, 2016; Coriale et al. 2013; CAMH, 2016).

PARTIAL FETAL ALCOHOL SYNDROME (pFAS)

This was previously, known as atypical FAS in the 1997 edition of the "4-Digit Diagnostic Code." People with pFAS have a confirmed history of prenatal alcohol exposure, but may lack growth deficiency or the complete facial stigmata. Central nervous system damage is present at the same level as FAS. These individuals have the same functional disabilities but "look" less like FAS (Streissguth, 1997; Oba, 2007).

FETAL ALCOHOL SYNDROME (FAS)

This subject term, the Fetal Alcohol Syndrome, can now be well described as follows: A British parliamentary report in 1834 on the

'Effects of Drunkenness on the Nation' indicated that some of the children of the drunkards tend to be 'born starved, shriveled and imperfect form' (NOFAS-UK, 2016). However, the earliest recorded observation of possible links between maternal alcohol use and Fetal damage was made in 1899 by Dr. William Sullivan, a Liverpool prison physician who noted higher rates of stillbirth in 120 alcoholic female prisoners than their sober female relatives. He suggested the causal agent to be alcohol use. This contradicted the predominating belief at the time that heredity caused intellectual disability, poverty, and criminal behavior. Anecdotal accounts of prohibitions against maternal alcohol use from biblical, ancient Greek, and ancient Roman sources imply a historical awareness of links between maternal alcohol use and negative child outcomes. For example, in the Bible, Judges 13:4 (addressed to a woman who was going to have a baby) read thus: "Therefore be careful and drink no wine or strong drink, and eat nothing unclean" (ESV).

In 1725, British physicians petitioned the House of Commons on the effects of strong drink when consumed by pregnant women saying that such drinking is "…too often the cause of weak, feeble, and distempered children, who must be, instead of an advantage and strength, (but rather) a charge to their country." Moreover, in Gaelic Scotland, mothers and nurses were not, allowed to consume ale during pregnancy and breastfeeding. Claims that alcohol consumption caused idiocy were part of the Teetotalism's message in the 19th century, but such claims, despite some attempts to offer evidence, were ignored because no mechanism could be advanced (NOFAS-UK, 2016; Streissguth, 1997; Oba, 2007; Jackson, 1828; Jonathan, 1870; Tait 2010; Sullivan, 1899).

Fetal Alcohol Syndrome which is presently regarded as the most severe of all the alcohol associated birth defects was named in 1973 by two dysmorphologists, Drs. Kenneth Lyons Jones and David Weyhe Smith of the University of Washington Medical School in Seattle, United States. They identified a pattern of "craniofacial, limb, and cardiovascular defects associated with prenatal growth and developmental delay" in eight unrelated children of three ethnic groups, all born to mothers who were alcoholics. The pattern of malformations indicated that the damage was prenatal. However, news of the discovery shocked some, while others were skeptical of the findings. Earlier, Paul Lemoine of Nantes, France, had already published a study in a French medical journal in 1968, about children with distinctive features whose mothers were alcoholics, and in the US, Christy Ulleland and colleagues at the University of Washington Medical School had conducted an 18-month study in 1968–1969 documenting the risk of maternal alcohol consumption among the offspring of 11 alcoholic mothers. The Washington and Nantes findings were confirmed by a research group in Gothenburg, Sweden, in 1979. Researchers in France, Sweden, and the United States were struck by how similar these children looked, though they were not related, and how they behaved in the same unfocused and hyperactive manner. Within nine years of the Washington discovery, animal studies, including that of monkey carried out at the University of Washington Primate Centre by Sterling Clarren, had confirmed that alcohol was a teratogen. By 1978, 245 cases of FAS had been reported by medical researchers. Prior to Fetal alcohol syndrome being specifically identified and named in 1973, only a few studies had noted differences between the children of mothers who used alcohol during pregnancy or breast-feeding and those who did not, and identified alcohol use as a possible contributing factor rather than heredity (Streissguth, 1997; Jones et al., 1973; Streissguth, 2002; Lemoine 1968; Ulleland, 1972; Olegard, 1979; Clarren, 2005).

While many syndromes are eponymous, that is, named after the physician first reporting the association of symptoms, David Weyhe Smith altruistically named FAS after the causal agent of the symptoms. He reasoned that doing so would encourage prevention, believing that if people knew maternal alcohol consumption caused the syndrome, then abstinence during pregnancy would follow from patient education and public awareness. At the time, nobody was aware of the full range of possible birth defects from FAS or its rate of prevalence (Olegard, 1979).

DISTINGUISHING FETAL ALCOHOL SYNDROME

Moreover, it is now well known that the efforts of identifying FAS children require the assistance of combined team of medical professionals, therapists, educators and social workers. Although FAS can be recognized from birth, but most of the characteristic features are expressed between 8 months and 8 years of life. The risk for potential Fetal alcohol syndrome could be established during the first prenatal visit. Prenatal indicators for potential alcohol use would note smaller than expected growth in length, weight, and head measurements. Slower than expected head growth is a reflection of subnormal brain growth. Once born, the above-noted facial changes will lead the pediatrician to consideration of the diagnosis of FAS. In addition, an individual with FAS may experience a lifelong litany of both physical and intellectual challenges (Clinical Growth Chart Archived, 2010; FAS facial features Archived, 2007; Lang, 2006).

To establish the diagnosis of Fetal alcohol syndrome, specific criteria must be met. These include documentation of the followings:

- characteristic craniofacial abnormalities
- smaller than expected prenatal and/or postnatal growth parameters
- central nervous system abnormalities.
- history of maternal ante/prenatal alcoholism
  (Astley, 2004; Malbin, 2002; Rasmussen et al., 2016)

Most of the available features of FAS may or may not be present in a given child. However, the most common and consistent features of FAS involve the followings:

1) *Unique facial characteristics:* a thin upper lip; a uniquely smooth ridge between the upper lip and nose – the philtrum; and a smaller than normal space between the upper and lower eyelids - short palpebral fissure;

2) *Growth delay:* smaller than expected length, weight, and head circumference measurements during both intrauterine and post-birth growth;

3) *Central nervous system abnormalities:* (a) structural - small brain size and slower than expected growth; (b) functional - global developmental delay in motor skills, language acquisition and utilization, problems with attention hyperactivity, social skill deficiencies, etc. (Clinical growth charts, 2007; Coriale et al., 2013; Malbin, 2002).

These features are, usually expressed in the following: Birth weight and growth is diminished. Retardation of longitudinal growth is evident on the measurements of length in infancy and of standing height later in childhood. The growth lag is permanent and performance is impaired. The FAS infant is irritable. The older FAS child is hyperactive. Fine motor skills are impaired with weak grasp, poor hand-eye coordination, and tremors with low intelligence. The average IQ is in the 60s. The head is small (microcephalic). This decrease may not even be apparent to family and friends. It is evident upon comparison of the child's head circumference to that of a normal child on a growth chart. The usual degree of microcephaly in FAS is, classified as mild to moderate. It is primarily due to failure of brain growth. The consequences are neither mild nor moderate. The face is characteristic with short eye openings (palpebral fissures), sunken nasal bridge, short nose, flattening of the cheek bones and midface, smoothing and elongation of the philtrum and smooth, thin upper lip. The skeleton shows characteristic changes; abnormal position and function of joints, shortening of the metacarpal bones leading to the fourth and fifth fingers, and shortening of the distal phalanx in the fingers. There is also a small fifth finger nail and a single transverse (simian) crease across the palm. A heart murmur is often, heard and then may go away. The basis is usually a hole between the right and left sides of the heart, between the ventricles or less commonly, the atria. A number of other birth defects can occur in children with FAS. These include such major birth deformities as hydrocephalus, cleft lip and sometimes with a cleft palate, coarctation of the aorta, and meningomyelocele (Lang, 2006; FADP – Fetal Alcohol Diagnostic Program (2007).

The expression of FAS features changes from birth to adulthood. From age 0-5 years, there is growth retardation, poor sleep/wake cycle, behavioral difficulty in attention and adapting to changes. Age 6-10 years is characterized by learning, understanding and cognitive impairments. If unchecked, at adolescent and adulthood, these difficulties could lead to secondary obvious disabilities like mental health disorders, substance abuse and other behavioral and societal menace, which result from the neuro development deficit (FADP – Fetal Alcohol Diagnostic Program, 2007).

Until lately, the establishment of precise and uniform delineating diagnostic criteria for FAS had remained a herculean task in particular to delineate the features from the other related conditions of birth defects resulting from alcoholism; since there was until recently none yet any available standard clinical diagnostic test but only rely on observable features. To this end, a Committee on Identification of FAS was set up in the United States, to avoid controversies; it was to bring out such diagnostic yardstick that will be consistent and accurate and be available and useful in exactly the same way by everyone. This must meet two evaluating requirements, which are thus: reliability – a measure of precision, and validity – the clinical relevance. These will make the diagnosis stable, and consistent over time and agreeable among clinicians and other concerned parties to make precisely the same diagnosis from anywhere even with time gaps between the assessment and the absence of information about previous clinicians' verdict. With this idea, nosologists have reached concession for a reliability coefficient on a scale level of 0.5 to 0.6 and validity of 0.7 to 0.9 in respect of these diagnostic criteria; bearing in mind that attempts to set FAS diagnostic criteria must swing between two ends - narrow and broad; this means to be narrow as to improve reliability, precision, and at the same time be broad to enhance generalization. The narrow-window criterion would be applied in research while the broad for clinical studies. The idea behind this was that if such FAS diagnosis is developed, it can also be used in the training of more clinicians working in this field. However, the followings are yet among the points that were being considered whether to be included in the criteria for diagnosis by the Committee on Identification of FAS, that is, history of the mothers' drinking habits and the physical, behavioral and cognitive features of FAS patients. It is yet under consideration if the designed criteria could be used across the life span of the FAS victims (Diagnosis and clinical evaluation of FAS, Institute of Medicine, 1996; Bertrand et al., 2004).

Presently, differential diagnosis of FAS is still a challenge. The development of diagnostic criteria should hence, also include the biomarkers to detect children at risk and enhance early interventions. This will also define the behavioral, physical and genetic factors for better clinical management of FAS. So far, FAS clinical examination is presently based on a 4-digit diagnostic coding in observable deficits in the following four features, that is, growth, craniofacial, brain and maternal alcoholism. Diagnostic evaluation in each criterion is then scored corresponding points as follow: absent or unlikely – 1; probable or unknown – 2; possible or likely – 3; and definite or present – 4. The code 4/4/4/4 for instance, indicates complete picture and is diagnostic of the Fetal Alcohol Syndrome (Diagnosis and clinical evaluation of FAS, Institute of Medicine, 1996; Bertrand et al., 2004).

CONCLUSION

The US Congress in 2002 tasked the Centre for Disease Control and Prevention (CDC), National Centre for Birth Defects and Developmental Disabilities (NCBDDD) and the National Task Force on Fetal Alcohol Syndrome and Fetal Alcohol Effect (NTFFAS/FAE) to develop comprehensive diagnostic criteria. This Committee in partnership with a Scientific Working Group (SWG) of experts in FAS research came out with a consensus "Fetal Alcohol Syndrome: Guideline for Referral and Diagnosis" within two years period and harmonized it with other existing diagnostic systems. This had since then provided a scientific state-of-the-art guideline for standard diagnostic criteria of FAS, which is useful to clinicians, scientists and other service providers. The guideline, for instance, indicates FAS distinct diagnostic features which distinguish FAS from the other similar alcohol related congenital defects acronyms or terminologies that were described earlier in this chapter. Moreover, currently, FAS is the only expression of prenatal alcohol exposure defined by the International Statistical Classification of Diseases and Related Health Problems and had been assigned ICD-9 and diagnoses (Bertrand et al., 2004).

REFERENCES

[1]   Aase J. M., Jones K. L. and Clarren S. K. (1995). "Do we need the term FAE?" *Paediatrics*. 95(3): 428–430. PMID7862486.

[2]   Abel, E. L., Jacobson S. and Sherwin B. T. (1983). "*In utero* alcohol exposure: Functional and structural brain damage." *Neurobehavioural Toxicology and Teratology*. 5(3): 363–366. PMID68 77477.

[3]   Adebisi, S. S. (2002). *Teratogenic effects of ethanol-induced folic acid deficiency on the developing bones of Wistar rat foetuses.* Unpublished PhD Thesis. Ahmadu Bello University, Zaria, Nigeria.

[4]   *Alcohol guidelines review* (2016). Report from the guidelines development group to the UK Chief Medical officers, Department of Health.

[5]   *Antenatal Care for Uncomplicated pregnancies* (2017). NCE Clinical guidelines.

[6]   Astley, S. J. and Clarren, S. K. (1996). "Most FAS children have a smaller brain than other children. A case definition and photographic screening tool for the facial phenotype of Fetal alcohol syndrome." *Journal of Paediatrics*. 129(1): 33–41. doi: 10.1016/s0022-3476 (96) 70187-7. PMID8757560.

[7]   Astley, S. J. (2004). *Diagnostic Guide for Fetal Alcohol Spectrum Disorders: The 4-Digit Diagnostic Code.* Seattle: University of

Washington. PDF available at FAS Diagnostic and Prevention Network. Retrieved on 2007-04-11.

[8]   Astley, S. J., Stachowiak, J., Clarren, S.K. and Clausen, C. (2002). "Application of the Fetal alcohol syndrome facial photographic screening tool in a foster care population." *Journal of Paediatrics.* 141 (5): 712–717. doi: 10.1067/mpd.2002.129030. PMID12410204.

[9]   Bertrand, J., Floyd, R. L., Weber, M. K., O'Connor, M., Riley, E. R., Johnson, K. A. and Cohen, D. E. (2004) National Task Force on FAE/FAS. *Fetal Alcohol Syndrome: Guidelines for Referral and Diagnosis* (PDF). Centre for Disease Control and Prevention.

[10] Blackburn L., (2009). *Facing the challenge and shaping the future for primary and secondary aged students with Fetal Alcohol Spectrum Disorders (FAS-eDProject) Literature Review*, National Organisation for Fetal Alcohol Syndrome- UK.

[11] Braton, R. (1996). *Fetal Alcohol Syndrome: how you can help prevent it.* Postgraduate Medical Education, 98(5): 197-200.

[12] Brent, Q. H. (1973). Alcohol related illnesses. In: *Drug abuse: Psycology, Sociology, Pharmacology.* Brigham Young. University Press. Provo, pp. 191 – 200.

[13] CAMH (2016). *More than 400 conditions co-occur with Fetal Alcohol Spectrum Disorders (FASD), CAMH study finds.* www. camh.ca.

[14] Chudley, S. (2016). *Fetal alcohol spectrum disorder: Canadian guidelines for diagnosis.* CMAJ.172 (5 Suppl): S1–S21. doi: 10.1503/cmaj.1040302. PMC557121. PMID15738468.

[15] Clarren, S. (1988). *FAS: a diagnosis for two. Finding common ground: working together for the future.* British Columbia.

[16] Clarren, S. K. and Smith D. W. (1978). "Fetal alcohol syndrome." *New England Journal of Medicine.* 298 (19): 1063–1067. doi: 10.1056/NEJM197805112981906. PMID347295.

[17] Clarren, S. K. (2005). A thirty year journey from tragedy to hope. Foreword to Buxton, B. (2005). *Damaged Angels: An Adoptive Mother Discovers the Tragic Toll of Alcohol in Pregnancy.* New York: Carroll & Graf. ISBN0-7867-1550-2.

[18] *Clinical growth charts.* (2010). Retrieved at the Wayback Machine. National Center for Growth Statistics.

[19] Coles, C., Brown, R., Smith, I., Platzman, K., Erickson, S. and Falek A. (1991). "Effects of prenatal alcohol exposure at school age. Physical and cognitive development." *Neurotoxicol Teratol.* 13 (4): 357–67. doi: 10.1016/0892-0362(91)90084-A. PMID1921915.

[20] Committee to Study Fetal Alcohol Syndrome, Division of Bio-behavioral Sciences and Mental Disorders, Institute of Medicine (2016). *Fetal alcohol syndrome: diagnosis, epidemiology, prevention, and treatment.* Washington, D. C: National Academy Press. ISBN: 0-309-05292-0. Archived from the original on 11 March 2016.

[21] Coriale, G., Fiorentino, D., Di Lauro, F., Marchitelli, R., Scalese, B., Fiore, M., Maviglia, M., and Ceccanti, M., (2013). "Fetal Alcohol Spectrum Disorder (FASD): neurobehavioral profile, indications for diagnosis and treatment." *Rivista di psichiatria.* 48 (5): 359–69. doi: 10.1708/1356.15062. PMID24326748.

[22] Diagnosis and clinical evaluation of FAS. Institute of Medicine. (1996). *FAS Diagnosis, Epidemiology, prevention and Treatment.*

[23] Di Bartolo, I. and Carlos, G. L. (1987). Alcoholic Embryo-foetus pathology. *Prensa. Med. Argent.* 74(8): 361-364.

[24] Fetal Alcohol Spectrum Disorders and their persisting Sequelae in Adult. (2000). *Life Dtsch Arztebl Int.* 105(4): 693-698.

[25] *FAS facial features* (2007). Archived at the Wayback Machine. FAS Diagnostic and Prevention Network, University of Washington.

[26] *Facts about FASDs.* (2015). Archived from the original on 23 May 2015.

[27] *FADP – Fetal Alcohol Diagnostic Program* (2007). Archived at the Wayback Machine.

[28] Goddard, H.H. (1912). *The Kallikak Family: A Study in the Heredity of Feeble-Mindedness.* New York: Macmillan.

[29] Jackson, R. (1828). Valpy, Abraham John, ed. "Considerations on the Increase of Crime, and the Degree of its Extent." *The Pamphleteer.* London: John Hatchard and Son 29 (57): 325. OCLC1761801.

[30] Jennifer, L. T. (2010). *The Poisoned Chalice* (Tuscaloosa, AL: University of Alabama Press, 27, 28.

[31] Jonathan T. C. (1870). *Arts of Intoxication: The Aim and the Results.* New York Carlton & Lanahan, P. 173-175.

[32] Jones K. L.; Smith D. W. (1973). "Recognition of the Fetal alcohol syndrome in early infancy." *Lancet.* 2 (7836): 999–1001. doi: 10.1016/s0140-6736(73)91092-1. PMID4127281.

[33] Jones K., Smith, D. (1975). "The Fetal alcohol syndrome." *Teratology.* 12 (1): 1–10. doi: 10.1002/tera.1420120102.PMID116 2620.

[34] Lang, J. (2006). "Ten Brain Domains: A Proposal for Functional Central Nervous System Parameters for Fetal Alcohol Spectrum Disorder Diagnosis and Follow-up" (PDF). *Journal of the FAS Institute.* 4: 1–11. Archived (PDF).

[35] Lemoine, P., Harousseau, H., Borteyru, J. B. and Menuet J. C. (1968). "Les enfants de parents alcooliques. Anomalies observées, à propos de 127 cas." *Quest Medical.* 21: 476–482. Reprinted in PMID 12657907. ["Children of alcoholic parents. Observed anomalies, about 127 cases."]

[36] Malbin, D. (2002). *Fetal Alcohol Spectrum Disorders: Trying Differently Rather Than Harder.* Portland, OR: FASCETS, Inc. ISBN: 0-9729532-0-5.

[37] Malbin, D. (1993). *Fetal Alcohol Syndrome, Fetal Alcohol Effects: Strategies for Professionals.* Center City, MN: Hazelden. ISBN: 0-89486-951-5.

[38] Maternal alcohol intake prior to and during pregnancy and risks of adverse birth out comes (2014). Evidence from a British cohort. *J. Epidemiol. Community Health*; 68(6): 542-9.

[39] NOFAS-UK (2016). National Organisation for Fetal Alcohol Syndrome-UK. *Alcohol and pregnancy, prevention and management of fetal alcohol spectrum disorders.* British Medical Association.

[40] Oba, P.S. (2007). "History of FASD." *FAS Aware UK.* Archived from the original on 2017-01-04. Retrieved 2016-11-20.

[41] Olegard, R., Sabel, K. G., Aronsson, M. S., Johannsson. P. R., Carlsson C., Kyllerman, M., Iversen, K. and Hrbek A. (1979). "Effects on the child of alcohol abuse during pregnancy." *Acta Paediatrica Scandinavica.* 275: 112–121. PMID291283.

[42] Poskit, E. M. E. (1984). *Fetal Alcohol Syndrome. Alcohol and Alcoholism* 9 (2): 159 – 165.

[43] Rasmussen, C., Andrew, G., Zwaigenbaum, L., Tough, S. (2016). "Neuro behavioural outcomes of children with fetal alcohol spectrum disorders: A Canadian perspective." *Paediatrics & Child Health.* 13 (3): 185–191. ISSN1205-7088. PMC2529423 PMID19252695.

[44] Renwick, J., Asker, R. (1983). "Ethanol-sensitive times for the human conceptus." *Early Hum Dev.* 8 (2): 99–111. doi: 10.1016/ 0378-3782(83)90065-8. PMID6884260.

[45] Rosett, H., Weiner, L. and Edellin, K. (1981). Strategies for prevention of fetal alcohol effects. *J. American College of Obstetrics and Gynaecology.* 57 (1): 1-7.

[46] Smith, D. (1979) *The Fetal alcohol syndrome. Hospital practice.* P. 121-128.

[47] Smith, D. W. (1981). "Fetal alcohol syndrome and Fetal alcohol effects." *Neurobehavioral Toxicology and Teratology.* 3: 127.

[48] Streissguth, A. (1997). *Fetal Alcohol Syndrome: A Guide for Families and Communities.* Baltimore: Brookes Publishing. ISBN: 1-55766-283-5.

[49] Streissguth, A. P. Martin, D. C., Martin J. C., and Barr, H. M. (1981). The Seattle long prospective study on alcohol and pregnancy. *Neurol. Toxicol. Teratol.* 3: 223 – 233.

[50] Streisguth, A., Aase, J. and Claren, S. (1991). Fetal Alcohol Syndrome in adolescent and adults. *JAMA* 265(15): 1961-1967.

[51] Streissguth, A. P. (2002). In A. Streissguth, & J. Kanter (Eds.), *The Challenge in Fetal Alcohol Syndrome: Overcoming Secondary Disabilities.* Seattle: University of WA Press. ISBN: 0-295-97650-0.

[52] *Statistics on alcohol* (2005). The Health and Social Care Information Centre (HCSC) England.

[53] Sullivan, W. C. (1899). "A note on the influence of maternal inebriety on the offspring." *Journal of Mental Science*. 45 (190): 489–503. doi: 10.1192/bjp.45.190.489.

[54] Tait, J. L. (2010). *The Poisoned Chalice* (Tuscaloosa, AL: University of Alabama Press, 27, 28.

[55] Ulleland, C. N. (1972). "The offspring of alcoholic mothers." *Annals of the New York Academy of Sciences*. 197: 167–169. Bibcode: 1972NYASA.197.167U. doi: 10.1111/j.1749-6632.1972.tb28142.x.P MID4504588.

In: Fetal Alcohol Syndrome
Editor: Doug Knight

ISBN: 978-1-53614-602-8
© 2018 Nova Science Publishers, Inc.

Chapter 2

PRENATAL ALCOHOL EXPOSURE, BIOMARKERS AND FETAL ALCOHOL SPECTRUM DISORDERS

Paul R. Gard, PhD, Media Zanganeh and David J. Timson, PhD*

School of Pharmacy and Biomolecular Science,
University of Brighton, Brighton, UK

ABSTRACT

Fetal Alcohol Spectrum Disorders (FASD) is the term used to describe neurobehavioral disorders associated with prenatal alcohol exposure ranging from the most severe Fetal alcohol syndrome (FAS) with facial dysmorphology, through partial Fetal alcohol syndrome (pFAS) to alcohol-related birth defects (ARBD). Many of the cognitive impairments associated with FASD are similar to those seen in Attention Deficit Hyperactivity Disorder (ADHD), Autistic Spectrum Disorders and other such conditions. There are considerable problems in diagnosing FASD and evidence of more than minimal exposure to ethanol during

* Corresponding Author: P.R.Gard@brighton.ac.uk.

pregnancy is an important criterion. Information on the mother's alcohol consumption during pregnancy may not be available, or may be inaccurate. Furthermore, approximately half of children affected by FASD may not exhibit signs of CNS dysfunction until they are preschool or school-age when the child and the mother may have become separated.

Early accurate differential diagnosis would enable the most effective treatments to be used. Ideally biomarkers would be identified which would enable confirmation of prenatal alcohol exposure. The use of meconium as an accessible fetal source of fatty acid ethyl esters (FAEEs), ethyl glucuronide (EtG) and ethyl sulfate (EtS) is frequently considered, but this is only applicable for the first few days of the neonate's life. The use of neonatal blood phosphatidylethanol (PEth) has also been discussed, but again the longevity of this biomarker is short. More recently results from animal studies of neonatal plasma microRNA biomarkers and changes to histone modifications have provided new opportunities, and DNA methylation has been suggested as a potential biomarker. Our own work suggests that prenatal alcohol exposure may induce long-lived changes in brain derived neurotrophic factor (BDNF) and brain aminopeptidase activity which may be reflected in changes in plasma or urine.

In the light of the evidence that many fetuses are exposed to alcohol but do not exhibit any degree of FASD, this review will assess the evidence of reliability of emerging enduring markers of prenatal alcohol exposure and explore whether they correlate only with prenatal alcohol exposure or also with FASD.

INTRODUCTION

The Diagnostic and Statistical Manual of Mental Disorders (5ᵗʰ Edition, DSM-V) describes *Neurobehavioral Disorder Associated With Prenatal Alcohol Exposure* which is characterized by features such as impaired global intellectual performance, executive functioning, learning and memory. More commonly the term Fetal Alcohol Spectrum Disorders (FASD) is used to describe the neurobehavioral disorders associated with prenatal alcohol exposure ranging from the most severe Fetal alcohol syndrome (FAS) with its facial dysmorphology, through partial Fetal alcohol syndrome (pFAS) to alcohol-related birth defects (ARBD). Importantly, within DSM-V the first criterion for diagnosis of any of these disorders is 'more than minimal exposure to alcohol during gestation, including prior to pregnancy recognition'. It goes on to state that 'confirmation of gestational exposure to alcohol may be obtained from maternal self-report of alcohol use in pregnancy, medical or other records, or clinical observation', although it is accepted that presence of the features of full-blown FAS (e.g., facial dysmorphology and growth retardation) can be used as evidence of significant prenatal alcohol exposure.

Problems arise with these diagnostic criteria and guidelines, however, when FASD is not immediately suspected or the child and the mother become separated. DSM-V recognizes that approximately half of affected children may not exhibit signs of CNS dysfunction until they are preschool- or school-age and furthermore due to difficulties obtaining an accurate assessment of the cognitive abilities of very young children, 'it is appropriate to defer a diagnosis for children 3 years of age and younger'. Reliance of maternal self-report or clinical observations so long after the birth can be problematic.

A long-lived, reliable, specific marker of prenatal alcohol exposure, detectable in the child, would remove the need to contact or interview the biological mother or to consult contemporaneous clinical notes when considering a 'late' diagnosis if FASD. Furthermore differentiation from Attention Deficit Hyperactivity Disorder (ADHD), Autistic Spectrum Disorders, genetic conditions such as Williams's syndrome and Down syndrome and other teratogenic conditions would be possible, enabling the most appropriate treatment options to be explored.

PERIPHERAL MARKERS OF ALCOHOL USE

It is possible to detect alcohol in the body using multiple body fluids such as saliva, blood, urine and sweat. Typically the enzymes responsible for alcohol metabolism are saturated thus the metabolism is zero-order, at approximately 8g of alcohol per hour which causes limitations in detection time (Wolff and Marshall, 2006). There are, however a range of ethanol metabolites that can be measured, in a range of tissues. In adults, metabolites have been determined in blood, urine, hair and nails and much effort has been expended looking for markers of alcohol consumption in pregnant women and infants.

Gamma-Glutamyltransferase (GGT)

Chronic alcohol exposure causes an elevation in the enzyme γ-glutamyltransferase (GGT); however, only the hepatic isoform of GGT is identifiable in the blood. GGT is mostly used as a clinical marker of hepatic damage. Serum GGT levels may be elevated in response to various kinds of drugs, and therefore the specificity and sensitivity of GGT as a potential biomarker of chronic alcohol consumption are still under question (Joya et al., 2012). The half-life for the detection of elevated serum GGT is 14 to 21 days (Bakhireva and Savage, 2011).

Halmesmaki, Roine and Salaspuro (1992) analyzed serum and urine GGT in 25 pregnant women consuming 150 g of alcohol weekly (approximately 21 g/day, equivalent to 200ml table wine) and abstinent age-matched pregnant women. This study demonstrated that high GGT levels represented chronic alcohol consumption in pregnant women; however GGT is not specific for alcohol and can be altered by many physiological and pathological factors such as atrial fibrillation (Lee et al., 2017), diabetic nephropathy (Carvalho et al., 2011), endometrial cancer (Seebacher et al., 2012), hypertension (Lee et al., 2002), gestational diabetes (Koenig and Seneff, 2015) and the use of enzyme-inducing or enzyme-inhibiting drugs.

Franzini et al. (2013) studied four fractions of GGT in the human plasma in alcoholic participants, participants who were abstinent for one month and non-drinkers. Abstainers and alcohol-dependent participants had significantly higher serum GGT levels than the control group. The s-fraction of GGT was of particular interest, as there was a 13.1 fold increase in its levels in the serum in alcohol-dependent participants. Furthermore, participants who were abstinent for a month prior to the study had a decrease in total serum GGT levels, where f-GGT and b-GGT fractions returned to their normal levels, and s-GGT and m-GGT values remained consistently high. Analyzing GGT fractions in the plasma rather than total serum GGT may lead to an increase in the specificity of this enzyme as a potential biomarker of alcohol consumption (Franzini et al., 2013) but the GGT fractions have not yet been determined in children exposed to alcohol in utero.

Carbohydrate-Deficient Transferrin (CDT)

Carbohydrate-deficient transferrin is a modified form of iron transporter protein transferrin, and another serum biomarker of chronic alcohol consumption. The detection window of serum CDT is 2 to 4 weeks after alcohol consumption (Bakhireva and Savage, 2011; Crunelle et al., 2016). One hundred male patients with known or suspected history of alcohol-dependence were tested for CDT as a potential biomarker of chronic alcohol consumption. The participants had a history of consuming 105 ± 94.7 g/day of ethanol, which is significantly higher than the 60 g/day (equivalent to 600ml Table wine) associated with the development of cirrhosis in males; the results of this study demonstrated a significant correlation between CDT and the reported daily alcohol consumption (Golka et al., 2004).

Throughout the normal gestational period, total transferrin levels increase which has led to CDT being measured as a fraction of total transferrin (% CDT). In 2011, Kenan et al. analyzed alterations to serum transferrin glycosylation during pregnancy and the potential effects of these changes on the reliability of using serum % CDT as a marker of alcohol consumption in this period. 24 pregnant women participated in this study and donated serum samples during the pregnancy and at 8 weeks (or longer) after delivery. Gradually increasing changes in transferrin microheterogeneity, different to the expected changes as a result of excessive alcohol use were observed throughout the gestational period. Throughout the third trimester of pregnancy, an increase in % disialotransferrin (the main focus of % CDT analysis) was observed in approximately 40% of the pregnant women. CDT is therefore unreliable as a measure of alcohol intake during pregnancy (Kenan et al., 2011), and has not been assessed as a potential biomarker in neonates or infants.

Phosphatidylethanol (PEth)

Another potential biomarker for alcohol use is phosphatidylethanol (PEth). PEth is an abnormal phospholipid developed in the presence of phosphatidylcholine, phospholipase D and ethanol in the erythrocyte membrane (Bracero et al., 2017). According to *in vitro* studies of whole human erythrocytes, incubation with ethanol for a period of 24 hours leads to the formation of PEth in the blood; the quantity of PEth formed is also directly proportional to the amount of alcohol present (Viel et al., 2012). In 2000, Varga et al. analysed blood PEth of fifteen alcoholic patients. They discovered that the half-life of blood PEth is 4 days, and its detection window is 2 weeks (Varga et al., 2000). In 2012, Kwak et al. analyzed blood PEth in pregnant women in their first trimester who reported consuming alcohol during pregnancy, and age-matched abstinent pregnant women also in their first trimester who reported no alcohol consumption for 6 months prior to conception. According to this team, due to the direct dependency of PEth development on alcohol, the specificity of this metabolite as a biomarker is theoretically 100%. None of the abstinent pregnant women in the study (n = 26) showed quantifiable levels of blood PEth; however, the range of PEth concentration in pregnant women who consumed low to moderate levels of alcohol 4 to 6 weeks before sample collection was between 4.8 nmol/L and 212.5 nmol/L and clearly distinguishable from the control group. This team demonstrated the specificity of PEth and the reliability of its use as a potential biomarker to detect alcohol consumption during pregnancy by distinguishing between pregnant women with previous low to moderate drinking behavior (up to 4 weeks prior to testing) and abstinent pregnant women (Kwak et al., 2012).

Bakhireva et al. (2013 or 2014?) analyzed the validity of using PEth in dried blood spot (DBS) cards of neonates as a potential screening method of prenatal alcohol exposure. Pregnant women who were included in the study group reported consuming either 3 or more drinks per week, or at least one incident of binge-drinking behavior per week during pregnancy? The results of this study demonstrated the ability of PEth-DBS to identify prenatal alcohol exposure. The authors speculated that blood collected at the time of the routine neonatal heel puncture could be used as a routine screen of prenatal alcohol exposure (Bakhireva et al., 2014).

Ethyl Glucuronide and Ethyl Sulfate

Ethyl glucuronide (EtG) and ethyl sulfate (EtS) are minor alcohol metabolites; the former is formed by the conjugation of ethanol and glucuronic acid, and the latter is formed by the conjugation of ethanol and a sulfate group. A study in 2004 (Dresen, Weinmann and Wurst, 2004) investigated urinary EtG and EtS levels as potential biomarkers of alcohol consumption. According to this study, EtS and EtG had similar detection times and could be identified in the urine for up to 26 hours after alcohol consumption (Data from (Bakhireva and Savage, 2011) suggesting that the detection time for urinary EtG is longer than EtS, and closer to 3-5 days); ethanol is present in urine for up to 10 hours after consumption. Dresen, Weinmann and Wurst also reported the absence of EtG and EtS in the urine of volunteers after one week of abstinence, making these biomarkers highly specific (Dresen, Weinmann and Wurst, 2004). Based on the detection time of EtG and EtS in the urine, however, we can conclude that these metabolites would not be useful tools in identifying prenatal alcohol exposure using neonatal urine; this is due to the fact that urinary EtG and EtS cannot paint an accurate picture of maternal drinking behavior throughout pregnancy, from the time of conception until delivery. This short detection window limits our knowledge on maternal drinking behavior to only approximately 30 hours before testing. Furthermore, urinary tract infections (UTIs) are a common occurrence in pregnant women, and the hydrolysis of EtG by some strains of Escherichia coli possessing β-glucuronidase activity in individuals with UTIs can lead to falsely negative results (Kissack, Bishop and Roper, 2008).

Fatty Acid Ethyl Esters (FAEEs)

FAEEs are primarily formed by non-oxidative enzymatic esterification of ethanol with free serum fatty acids; an increase in serum FAEEs is directly proportional to an increase in alcohol intake in individuals and FAEEs have previously been found in the heart, brain, blood, liver and adipose tissue. Blood FAEEs are not ideal biomarkers of alcohol consumption due to their short half-life (approximately 24 hours after alcohol consumption); FAEEs can, however, be used as reliable biomarkers of alcohol exposure in other matrices (Littner and Bearer, 2007).

In the field of forensic toxicology, hair analysis is used to test for and detect a wide array of substances. Interestingly, hair ethyl oleate, ethyl stearate, ethyl palmitate and ethyl myristate are FAEEs used to detect chronic excessive alcohol consumption in the workplace, based on the European guidelines for workplace alcohol testing. Results can determine whether or not the donors consume over 60g of pure ethanol on a daily basis over the period of several months, as this amount is considered to be "chronic excessive alcohol drinking" by the World Health Organisation (Agius and Kintz, 2010). In a study by Pragst et al., hair samples from 21 deceased alcoholics were collected followed by post-mortem examination at a medical institute. Hair samples from 10 children and adult non-drinkers and 10 social drinkers were also collected for comparison. The results of this study revealed that the same four FAEES used to detect excessive alcohol consumption in the European guidelines for workplace alcohol testing were present in all the hair samples from alcoholic subjects. The concentrations of ethyl oleate and ethyl palmitate were the highest detected in the hair samples; the concentrations of the four FAEEs, however, varied considerably between the subjects. In terms of the social drinkers, only ethyl palmitate was present in all the hair samples, this was followed by ethyl oleate, ethyl stearate and ethyl myristate at just above the limits of quantification in only two samples. Interestingly, no FAEEs were detected in the hair samples of the children and the non-drinkers. Based on the results of this study, HFAEEs are appropriate biomarkers to detect alcohol intake and distinguish between chronic alcohol consumption, social drinking and abstinence (Pragst et al., 2001).

Hair Ethyl Glucuronide

In 2009, Morini et al. investigated the sensitivity and specificity of using hair EtG as a potential biomarker of chronic alcohol consumption. 98 subjects were recruited in the study ranging from non-drinkers to heavy drinkers, and a questionnaire was used to determine their alcohol consumption within the last 3 months and 2 weeks respectively; a 3 cm segment of hair was collected for analysis. This team decided upon a 27 pg/mg cut-off concentration for hair EtG (HEtG), higher than previous studies, to avoid achieving a lower sensitivity and specificity of detection. Based on the results of this study, HEtG is more reflective of alcohol consumption in the last 3 months in comparison to the last 2 weeks, which may be due to the 3 cm hair segment used, where on average each centimeter of hair has grown over a month. Despite the lack of a strong correlation between HEtG and alcohol consumption over a period of 3 months, a general positive correlation can be determined (Morini, Politi and Polettini, 2009).

The same group also determined that the minimum amount of neonatal hair required for testing for HEtG is 30 to 50 mg, and the 4 to 12 mg hair samples collected from newborns in their study were not enough to test for HEtG reliably; this was due to the sparseness of neonatal hair. HEtG is therefore not a useful marker of prenatal alcohol exposure in neonates (Morini et al., 2010).

In a recent study Cappelle and colleagues studied EtG levels in nails as well as hair as potential markers of alcohol consumption. Nail and hair samples were collected from participants undergoing treatment at two psychiatric centers for alcohol use disorders. Interestingly, this team found a significant correlation between HEtG and fingernail and toenail EtG (Cappelle et al., 2017). It is possible that this can be a very useful tool in identifying prenatal alcohol exposure in neonates if studied further, as fetal fingernails develop at approximately the 12th week of pregnancy, and can be representative of Fetal environment during that period.

The biological matrix that has produced the most reliable biomarkers of prenatal alcohol exposure is meconium. Meconium is the earliest feces of the neonate, replaced by normal feces 2-4 days after the commencement of feeding. In 2006, Ostrea et al. analyzed the meconium of 124 children to determine the specificity of fatty acid ethyl esters (FAEEs, see above) as potential biomarkers of prenatal alcohol exposure. The researchers proposed that the presence of these FAEEs in the meconium of the alcohol-exposed group was a result of the esterification of docosahexanoate acid (DHA) and α-linolenic acid by ethanol, leading to their excretion as soluble ethyl esters and limiting their availability for normal Fetal development. They interviewed 124 pregnant women regarding the degree of their alcohol consumption at the time of conception and throughout the gestational period; to account for under-reporting due to the social stigma surrounding risky behaviors during pregnancy, the drinking amount at the time of conception was used as the measure of usual alcohol intake. Standard alcohol-use questionnaires were also used to gain a better understanding of the range of alcohol consumption in the alcohol-exposed group. Of the FAEEs detected in the meconium, ethyl linoleate and ethyl arachidonate (AA) in particular demonstrated high specificity for identifying prenatal alcohol exposure in neonates. Despite the fact ethyl linoleate was unable to determine the level of prenatal alcohol exposure accurately (sensitivity), its specificity (i.e., ability to identify any alcohol exposure) was very high; thus identification of ethyl linoleate in the meconium is very likely to be evidence of prenatal alcohol exposure.

Similarly, ethyl AA and ethyl DHA have low sensitivity as potential biomarkers of prenatal alcohol exposure, but high specificity and are therefore also highly indicative of prenatal alcohol exposure if detected in the meconium. Ethyl DHA is of particular interest, as DHA is crucial for normal fetal brain and retinal development thus excretion of ethyl DHA may be an important factor in developing FASD through interference with normal brain development. Its presence may therefore be indicative not only for prenatal alcohol exposure, but also for FASD (Ostrea et al., 2006).

Another study in 2003 highlighted the importance of FAEE detection in the meconium in regards to the prevalence of FASD in two geographically and culturally different populations in the US. This study focused on detecting a wide range of FAEEs (palmitoleic, palmitic, linoleic, oleic, stearic and arachidonic acid ethyl esters) in the meconium of 436 neonates from Hawaii, as well as 289 neonates in Utah. According to this team, 16.7% of the neonates in the Hawaii and 12.1% of the neonates in Utah were exposed to alcohol prenatally (FAEES > 50 ng/g). These figures were both in line with the prevalence of prenatal alcohol exposure in the two regions; the former is based on maternal interviews and the latter is due to a lower rate of adult alcohol consumption in the region. The results of this study are also in part in line with the later findings of Ostrea et al., where 90% of the samples in Hawaii and more than 80% of the samples in Utah considered "positive" for FAEEs contained ethyl linoleate, making it particularly promising as a potential biomarker of prenatal alcohol exposure; this was closely followed by ethyl oleate (51% and 65% respectively). However, this study differs from the study by Ostrea et al. in that no ethyl AA was detected in the meconium; stability testing revealed that ethyl AA is highly susceptible to degradation from heat and light, and the best way to store FAEEs is to freeze them within 12 hours (Bakhireva and Savage, 2011) and if necessary, transport them in a dark environment and on ice. If these storage conditions are met, only 11% of total FAEEs will be lost over 6 days, compared to storage at room temperature and exposure to light where 86% of the total FAEEs can be lost within 24 hours (Moore et al., 2003).

It is crucial to validate the specificity and accuracy of using FAEEs as potential biomarkers in prenatal alcohol exposure particularly. Bearer and colleagues recruited and interviewed 27 pregnant women of European, Khoi aboriginal, Malaysian and black African descent at an out-patient clinic in South Africa regarding their daily alcohol consumption; the interviews took place at recruitment, at an antenatal visit, and one month postpartum. FAEEs were then analyzed in random meconium samples obtained from the infants' diapers. According to the results of this study, similar to data reported by Moore and colleagues, ethyl oleate concentration was positively correlated with prenatal alcohol exposure to 3 or more standard alcohol units per day. Interestingly, several studies from the USA have suggested that FASD's neurobehavioral and growth outcomes are associated with prenatal alcohol exposure to five or more standard alcohol units in one occasion (Streissguth et al., 1994; Jacobson et al., 1998); it can therefore be hypothesized that detecting FAEEs in the meconium has made it possible to identify prenatal alcohol exposure at levels where the adverse neurobehavioral outcomes of FASD are not present. Furthermore, this study revealed that knowledge of number of drinks per occasion (binge-behavior) during the pregnancy, is more indicative of prenatal alcohol exposure than knowledge of overall weekly alcohol units consumed. This is evident from the correlation of FAEEs in the meconium to the amount of alcohol consumption in one setting during the pregnancy; the detection of FAEEs in the meconium may be due to extended exposure to alcohol past a particular threshold, rather than occasional low-dose exposure which is likely to be rapidly metabolized (Bearer et al., 2003).

To understand the origin of meconium FAEEs and the role of the placenta, Chan et al. investigated the presence of FAEEs inside the maternal-placental-Fetal unit and possible mechanisms for FAEE metabolism. Based on the results of this study, FAEEs from the maternal circulation are metabolized by the placenta and not transferred to the fetus; therefore FAEEs detected in the meconium are probably produced by the fetus through ethanol exposure and metabolism, making them direct biomarkers of true prenatal alcohol exposure (Chan et al., 2004; Koren et al., 2002).

Despite many advantages of using meconium to study fetal environment throughout pregnancy, there are also disadvantages that are noteworthy. Meconium collection is a non-invasive process as it is routinely excreted and available from most neonates. It also costs approximately $200 to $400 (£150 to £300) to test the sample, which is reasonably cost-effective (Burd and Hofer, 2008). However, meconium testing overall is more problematic to process than blood or urine analysis. Meconium begins accumulating in the Fetal gut at around the 20th week of the gestational period, and full-term neonates usually pass meconium within the first 24-48 hours of life; however, babies born with low birth weight may pass meconium approximately 36 hours after birth, at which time sample collection may be missed. Furthermore, meconium is a complex and unfamiliar matrix and requires further extraction steps for analysis and more difficult confirmation assays compared to urine (Kwong and Ryan, 1997). It is also not feasible to screen the meconium of every neonate globally, especially considering the legal and ethical issues that may rise up if implemented universally (Lange et al., 2014). According to Bakhireva and Savage, meconium may be entirely unavailable in up to 10% of neonates, especially premature babies. The specimen must also be frozen at ultralow temperatures no longer than 12 hours after collection to avoid affecting FAEE levels (Bakhireva and Savage, 2011).

The exact stage of the pregnancy where meconium starts accumulating in the fetal gut is not fully understood; it could start as early as the 12th week or most likely as late as the 20th week of the gestational period. The potential for meconium components to act as biomarkers of prenatal alcohol exposure is therefore limited to the fetoplacental environment in the later stages of pregnancy; this is not representative of maternal drinking behavior in the first trimester, as some women change their drinking habits after confirmation of pregnancy. Furthermore, multiple cut-off values used in various studies to determine a "positive" finding of FAEEs in the meconium and the use of several different FAEEs has led to inconsistencies in the available literature in relation to prenatal alcohol exposure. Specifying a universal limit of detection, using a combination of two or more biomarkers (Burd and Hofer, 2008) and focusing on widely studied FAEEs in relation to prenatal alcohol exposure such as ethyl linoleate and ethyl oleate can result in a more accurate understanding of their specificity and sensitivity in detecting prenatal alcohol exposure. Currently, there is also lack of knowledge about the validity of FAEEs in detecting discontinued previous binge-drinking behavior and their ability to differentiate mild to moderate drinking behavior from absolute abstinence (Bakhireva and Savage, 2011; Viel et al., 2012).

In a comprehensive study in 2015, Himes and colleagues studied the sensitivity and specificity of meconium ethyl glucuronide and ethyl sulfate (EtG and EtS, see above) as potential biomarkers of prenatal alcohol exposure and compared their practicability to meconium FAEEs. This team measured EtG and EtS levels in the meconium in relation to maternal self-report of alcohol consumption at or after the 19th week of pregnancy, to account for potential variability in meconium-formation period between different participants. Detailed data on the amount and pattern of alcohol consumption was collected from pregnant women (n = 108) through structured interviews prior to sample collection. Interestingly, this team considered meconium EtG concentration of ≥ 30 ng/g the "gold standard" with the highest agreement with reported prenatal alcohol exposure on or after the 19th week of pregnancy, at 81.8% sensitivity and 75.2% specificity to maternal self-report of alcohol consumption; EtS concentration of ≥ 5 ng/g followed with 68.6% sensitivity and 73% specificity to self-reported alcohol consumption. The results of this study demonstrated that EtG was detected in more samples (65.4%) than EtS or FAEEs. There was also a significant relationship between meconium EtG concentration of ≥ 30 ng/g and self-reported alcohol consumption on or after the 19th week of pregnancy; this strong dose-concentration relationship suggests that EtG can be used as a reliable and accurate biomarker of increasing prenatal alcohol exposure throughout the gestational period. It is noteworthy, however, that genetic polymorphisms of UDP-glucuronosyltyransferases (UTG), drug metabolizing enzymes, and hepatic dysfunction from chronic alcohol intake may lead to decreased EtG formation, which can in turn lead to EtG-negative meconium samples (Himes et al., 2015).

Morini et al. (2010) analyzed meconium EtG and EtS as well as HEtG and hair ethyl sulfate (HEtS) in 99 pregnant women and their neonates after delivery, as potential markers of prenatal alcohol exposure; both hair (9 cm segments) and meconium samples were analyzed. Interestingly, HEtG was not detected above the set 3 pg/mg limit of quantification in any of the maternal hair samples; as it has been established that HEtG can be used to detect even moderate drinking behavior, these results may mean that HEtG is not a suitable marker of occasional or light daily alcohol consumption (Morini et al., 2010). This is in line with the findings of Politi and colleagues in that if a 5 pg/mg cut-off point is appropriate to detect $\geq$ 40 g/day of alcohol consumption, and a 4 pg/mg cut-off point is appropriate to detect $\geq$ 30 g/day of alcohol consumption (Politi et al., 2006), then the participants of the Morini et al. study would have had to hypothetically consume 20 g of alcohol per day for 6 month prior to hair sample collection for HEtG to be detected above the 3 pg/mg limit of quantification. These limits of quantification are therefore unrealistic in terms of the ability to detect mild alcohol consumption in pregnant women. More studies must be done to optimize the use of HEtG as a marker of alcohol use, by adjusting the limit of quantification of HEtG, whilst assessing changes in sensitivity and specificity as a result; currently, however, HEtG is not an appropriate biomarker in detecting mild and occasional drinking in pregnant women.

Similarly, Joya and colleagues recruited 80 pregnant women, applied a questionnaire regarding alcohol consumption and collected 9 cm long hair samples to account for drinking pattern in all three trimesters of pregnancy. The meconium of 80 neonates were collected after delivery and both meconium and maternal hair samples were analyzed. Interestingly, this team observed a significant correlation between maternal HEtG and meconium EtG concentrations, especially in the last trimester (hair segment of 0 to 3 cm). They also observed a significant correlation between meconium EtG concentrations and meconium FAEE concentrations. Furthermore, all of the 22 neonates from the 22 mothers with overall undetectable HEtG levels, also demonstrated undetectable meconium EtG. 90.9% of the neonates from the 22 mothers with HEtG levels of > 30 pg/mg in one or more hair sections tested positive for meconium EtG (concentration ranging between 6.7 ng/g and 452.9 ng/g). 88.9% of the neonates from the 36 mothers with HEtG levels of between 7 pg/mg and 30 pg/mg in one or more hair sections tested positive for meconium EtG (concentration ranging between 6.7 ng/mg and 210.9 ng/mg). This study has intelligibly demonstrated the efficacy and reliability of using both maternal HEtG and neonatal meconium EtG to identify prenatal alcohol exposure in the second and third trimester, revealing good specificity and sensitivity when used together; this has been done by using maternal HEtG as a marker of alcohol consumption as opposed to maternal self-report to avoid incidences of under-reporting (Joya et al., 2015).

The aforementioned biomarkers of alcohol consumption all come with a series of advantages and disadvantages. According to Howlett and colleagues, using a combination of biomarkers of prenatal alcohol exposure as well as maternal self-report is of clinical value and can aid diagnosis; however, no blood biomarker so far has been as accurate as self-reporting to identify alcohol exposure during pregnancy (Howlett et al., 2017). An ideal biomarker of prenatal alcohol exposure must also have longevity to be identified years after birth, in early or late childhood. Liver enzymes appear to be affected by various physiological and pathological factors and are currently not ideal biomarkers of prenatal alcohol exposure, especially after birth. Alanine aminopeptidase (ApN) in the urine, related to the nephrotoxic effects of alcohol-dependency, has also been found to be a good potential biomarker of chronic alcohol consumption (Taracha et al., 2004), but this will be discussed further, later.

ANIMAL MODELS

Many researchers have attempted to use animal models, particularly rats and mice, to explore the effects of maternal ethanol exposure on the unborn fetus (see Petrelli et al., 2018). In the current context the aim would be to identify some physical (e.g., biochemical or epigenetic) change that correlates with prenatal alcohol exposure or even a change indicative of neuronal damage and/or cognitive impairment. Such animal models have significant advantages over clinical studies in that they allow controlled exposure to ethanol, at fixed doses, at specific periods during pregnancy and in particular patterns (e.g., binge-drinking versus constant low-level). Animal studies also remove the confounding factors of socio-economic status, educational status, income, nutritional status, etc. seen in human populations. The animals used are typically of 'inbred' strains, generated by sibling mating, and are considered to be > 99% genetically identical with similar, and controlled, prior experiences and nutritional status. On the other hand, however, animal studies are potentially misleading because of the different rates of development of mice and humans. For example the mouse gestation period is 20 days and the pups are born blind and relatively undeveloped; development continues postnatally. Thus days 1 - 10 of a mouse pregnancy are generally seen as being equivalent to the human first trimester, days 11 - 20 are the equivalent of trimester 2 and post-natal days 1 - 10 are equivalent to trimester 3. Related to this, mice have the advantage of the first day of pregnancy being relatively easily defined by the presence of a vaginal plug, whilst the first day of pregnancy in humans is more difficult to time accurately other than retrospectively.

One big difference between humans and rodents is the way in which ethanol is distributed around the body and metabolized. For example, the body water content per kilogram of body weight is different which means that apparent volumes of distribution for ethanol are different. Apparent volume of distribution is an estimate of how widely the ethanol is distributed around the body, so for example if a woman was given 40g ethanol (40000mg), and the plasma alcohol concentration was found to be 1mg/ml it could be estimated that all of the ethanol had been distributed to a total volume of 40000ml (40 liters). 40 liters equates to total body water of a 66Kg female, thus it would be estimated that the ethanol had been distributed evenly across all of the body water. In reality the apparent volume of ethanol distribution in human females is 0.63 liters/kg, but in mice is 0.8 liters/kg (Cederbaum, 2013), thus for a given dose of ethanol (mg/kg), mice would have a lower plasma ethanol concentration than Humans. It is also known that mice metabolize and excrete ethanol more rapidly than humans (ibid.). Thus in mouse studies, the doses of ethanol administered seem unfeasibly large, but are aimed at achieving blood alcohol concentrations comparable to those seen in humans after ethanol consumption, for example 80 mg/dl, the legal limit for driving in the UK.

Consider the following two examples of typical ethanol dosing regimens in mice. Firstly, investigating the effects of acute high doses of ethanol administered orally (typically called 'binge drinking') Schambra et al., (2017) gave mice 2.4g/kg ethanol, twice, 4 hours apart, and reported peak blood alcohol concentrations of 104 mg/dl. For a 65kg Human, 2.4g/kg ethanol equates to approximately 1.5 liters of table wine in a single bout. Alternatively some researchers use an *ab libitum* dosing schedule, i.e., putting ethanol in the drinking water, as a model of chronic low dose exposure. An intake of approximately 10 g ethanol per Kg body weight per day in mice is required to give a peak blood alcohol concentration of 80 mg/l (Petrelli et al., 2018). 10 g ethanol per Kg bodyweight per day in mice would equate to 6.5 liters of table wine over 24 hours in a 65kg Human.

Notwithstanding the seemingly unfeasible doses of ethanol used and the differences between mice and Humans, animal models of prenatal alcohol exposure have generated invaluable data. A recent review of animal data by Petrelli et al. (2018) clearly demonstrates that high, acute doses of ethanol (two doses of 2.9g/kg) on gestational days 7, 8 or 9 (first trimester equivalent) result in the characteristic craniofacial changes of FAS, as does chronic lower dose ethanol exposure (20g/kg/day) from days 1 to 8. The situation changes, however, later in pregnancy. Lower dose, consistent, prenatal ethanol exposure (10 - 20g/kg/day) was seen to produce anxiety and depression-like symptoms and deficits of learning and memory, without the craniofacial changes. It is thus suggested that early binge drinking by the mother may result in the facial features of FAS, whilst later sustained lower dose prenatal ethanol exposure may result in the cognitive changes. It is for these later effects that a diagnostic marker is needed.

To return to the theme of this review, the diagnosis of *Neurobehavioral Disorder Associated With Prenatal Alcohol Exposure* requires evidence of 'more than minimal exposure to alcohol during pregnancy' but that the presence of the features of full-blown FAS (e.g., facial dysmorphology and growth retardation) can be used as evidence of significant prenatal alcohol exposure. Being that the craniofacial dysmorphology appears to be a consequence of first trimester, high dose, alcohol exposure, and that the facial dysmorphology is itself a diagnostic criterion, there seems that little would be gained by identification of a biomarker of early, high-dose prenatal alcohol exposure. Sustained and later, lower-dose alcohol exposure, however, has the potential to cause neurobehavioral disorders that may be confused with Attention Deficit Hyperactivity Disorder (ADHD) and Autistic Spectrum Disorders, and would therefore benefit most from a differential diagnostic aid.

One of the earliest references to possible peripheral markers of PAE was that of Gottesfeld and colleagues (e.g., Gottesfeld et al., 1990) who reported that exposure of pregnant mice to an *ad libitum* oral diet of 4.8% ethanol throughout pregnancy resulted in offspring which, at about 6 weeks of age, showed reduced responses to immune challenges and reduced noradrenaline concentrations and β-adrenoceptor density in the thymus and spleen, but not the heart. Whilst of limited value as a peripheral marker of PAE, parallels could be drawn with the work of Carstens et al., (1987) who measured lymphocyte β-adrenoceptor binding in depressed and non-depressed individuals and found a significantly decreased number of receptors in patients. Whether chronic alcohol exposure has any effect on lymphocyte β-adrenoceptor characteristics has never been explored, but there is evidence that changes in these characteristics induced by increased blood pressure in rats are long-lasting, well beyond the period of hypertension (Fukuda et al., 1985). Lymphocyte β-adrenoceptors may therefore be of interest as a proxy measure of prenatal alcohol exposure and worthy of further investigation.

The endogenous opioid met-enkephalin is another potential biomarker. Abate et al. (2017) dosed pregnant rats intragastrically (i.e., via a feeding tube) with an acute ethanol dose of 2 g/kg on days 17 - 20 of pregnancy. The gestation period for a rat is 21.5 days. The adolescent offspring were tested at 30 days of age, which is considered pre-pubertal. The ethanol exposed animals exhibited decreased rearing behavior, which is indicative of increased response to stress, and increased met-enkaphalin in several brain areas but not all. This finding is interesting in the light of the work of Banks et al. (2003) who studied the effects of ethanol consumption (5% in drinking water) in mice over 56 days. Met-enkephalin was measured in the brain and serum. Brain concentrations of Met-enkaphalin were increased in ethanol-consuming mice in comparison to controls after 7, 10, and 14 days of ethanol drinking. Values then declined below those of controls after days 28 days. There were no significant differences in serum met-enkephalin concentrations between ethanol-treated and control animals at any of the time points, even though in control animals there is a significant correlation between brain and serum met-enkephalin concentrations. This finding indicates that ethanol disrupts the brain-serum correlation for met-enkephalin concentration and therefore draws into question the utility of serum met-enkephalin as a potential enduring biomarker of prenatal ethanol exposure, although it may warrant further evaluation.

There is also a significant body of literature that indicates that prenatal alcohol exposure elevates oxidative stress (see Fontaine et al., 2016). Brocardo et al. (2017), for example, treated pregnant rats with ethanol, via drinking water, to give peak blood alcohol concentrations of 90 - 100 mg/dl. There were three experimental groups, rats receiving ethanol only for days 1-10 of gestation, those receiving ethanol for days 11 - 21 of gestation and those receiving ethanol on post-partum days 4- 1 0. Offspring were tested at 60 days of age when lipid peroxidation was assessed in several brain areas using formation of malondialdehyde (MDA). Those offspring exposed to ethanol during the second and third trimester equivalent were found to have evidence of oxidative damage (i.e., increased lipid peroxidation) in the hippocampus, thus demonstrating that prenatal ethanol exposure can have long-term consequences in the adult brain by dysregulation of its redox status, possibly by depletion of the antioxidant glutathione (Fontaine et al., 2016). Changes in redox status have previously been examined *in vivo* using measurement of F_2-isoprostanes in cerebrospinal fluid, plasma and urine (Milne et al., 2005). Elevations of F_2-isoprostanes have been shown in neurodegenerative disorders, pulmonary disease and kidney disease (ibid). Daily, moderate alcohol intake for three weeks has been shown to increase, albeit non-significantly, urinary F_2-isoprostanes (Beulens et al., 2008). The effects of maternal alcohol consumption on neonate plasma or urine F_2-isoprostanes may therefore be worthy of investigation.

Hormones of the Hypothalamic-Pituitary-Adrenal (HPA) axis have also been shown to be influenced by prenatal alcohol exposure. Xia et al. (2014) dosed pregnant rats orally with ethanol (4g/kg/day) from day 11 of pregnancy until delivery. The male offspring were then fed a high fat diet until postnatal week 16 when blood samples were taken for determination of adrenocorticotrophic hormone (ACTH) and corticosterone (the rat equivalent of human cortisol). The results indicated that both ACTH and corticosterone were significantly decreased, by about 30%, in the rats exposed to ethanol prenatally. This might suggest that components of the HPA may be suppressed in children exposed to ethanol in utero, although there is no clinical evidence that this is the case. Dysregulation of the HPA has also been implicated in the aetiology of depressive illness, albeit it in terms of hypersensitivity to stress (e.g., Quinn et al., 2018), which would be a confounding factor considering the fact that children with FASD are known to have poor impulse control. The value of HPA parameters as biomarkers of prenatal alcohol exposure is therefore probably low. Lecuyer et al. (2017) injected pregnant mice with ethanol (3g/kg/day) from gestational days 15 to 20. Placental growth factor (PLGF) was determined within the placental tissue: prenatal alcohol exposure was shown to significantly decrease placental PLGF. Similar determination of PLGF in placentae of women known to have consumed alcohol during pregnancy also demonstrated a decrease. The authors discussed the relationship between PLGF, Vascular Endothelial Growth Factor (VEGF) and vascularization of the brain, suggesting that the decreased PLGF was reflective of poor development of the brain vasculature. The authors speculate that measurement of PLGF in the placenta, umbilical cord blood or even neonatal blood may be a reliable indicator of pre-natal alcohol exposure. Only placental PLGF has yet been explored and the sensitivity and longevity of any changes in neonatal blood are as yet unknown.

There is also a body of literature concerning the effects of prenatal alcohol exposure on inflammatory mediators. Raineki et al. (2017), for example, dosed pregnant rats on gestational days 1-21 in a manner similar to that described for Brocardo et al. (2017) above (6.6% ethanol in drinking water). Biochemical parameters were determined on postnatal day 12. The results showed that pups exposed to ethanol prenatally had significantly (30%) elevated serum C-reactive protein, a non-specific hepatic protein marker of inflammation, infection and trauma. These results supported the previous findings of the same group in that they had previously reported elevated serum TNF-α, interleukin-13 and interferon-γ, all inflammatory mediators (cytokines), on post-natal day 8 which had returned to control values by post-natal day 22. Whilst interesting, the lack of specificity of inflammatory mediators as biomarkers, and their lability render them unlikely to be of value as enduring markers of prenatal alcohol exposure.

Our own recent research suggests that prenatal alcohol exposure may also induce long-lived changes in brain derived neurotrophic factor (BDNF). Changes in this parameter may be reflected by changes in plasma or serum. BDNF is a nerve growth factor important in neuronal development, neuronal repair and learning and memory. It is known to be elevated at times of stress and other forms of neuronal trauma (e.g., infection and inflammation). It has been speculated that a deficiency of BDNF may precipitate depressive illness due to an inability of repair the neuronal damage induced by chronic low-grade stress (e.g., Duman et al., 1997). Antidepressant drugs have been shown to elevate plasma and brain BDNF, and this has been proposed as their mechanism of action (ibid.). BDNF has also been shown to be decreased in dementia (Laske et al., 2007), and it has been proposed that elevation of BDNF by use of antidepressants may be of benefit in the management of dementia (Liu et al., 2014). Terasaki and Schwarz (2017) reported that prenatal exposure of rats to ethanol 2g/kg twice daily from gestational days 10 - 16, which resulted in a maternal blood alcohol concentration of 70 mg/dl, resulted in increased BDNF gene expression in the perirhinal area of the brain at 90 days of age. Our own data in mice, as yet unpublished, supports these findings in that prenatal exposure to ethanol (5%) via drinking water throughout pregnancy and until weaning resulted in significantly elevated BDNF in the cerebrocortex, cerebellum and hippocampus at 124 days of age. Such elevated brain BDNF may indicate a prolonged neurochemical response to the fetal neuronal trauma of the alcohol exposure. These findings should be viewed in the perspective of discussions of the correlation between brain and plasma or serum BDNF (Naegelin et al., 2018). Plasma or serum BDNF is routinely used as a proxy measure of brain BDNF in studies of depressive illness and the effects of antidepressant drugs (e.g., Sen et al., 2008) and Dementia (e.g., Lee et al., 2015). That plasma or serum BDNF is thus a potential enduring marker of prenatal alcohol exposure therefore warrants further investigation, although the specificity of the marker is questionable as plasma BDNF has been seen to be elevated 48 hours post-delivery in infants with neonatal opiate abstinence syndrome (Subedi et al., 2017) and other workers have suggested that prenatal alcohol exposure decreases brain expression of BDNF and its receptor (see Fontaine et al., 2016).

Our work has also highlighted another set of possible biomarkers. Our earlier research has demonstrated that angiotensin IV, a component of the renin-angiotensin system, is able to improve learning and memory in animal models (Golding et al., 2010). The renin-angiotensin system is typically regarded as being a peripheral quasi-endocrine system which controls blood pressure, fluid balance and thirst. The textbook example of its actions would be a decrease in haemoperfusion of the kidney due to decreased blood pressure or haemorrhage resulting in secretion of the enzyme renin by the juxtaglomerular apparatus. This enzyme catalyses the conversion of the circulating hepatic protein angiotensinogen to angiotensin I. Angiotensin I is subsequently converted to angiotensin II by angiotensin-converting enzyme (ACE) which is present in high concentrations in the pulmonary vasculature. Angiotensin II, acting via its AT_1 and AT_2 receptors then causes vasoconstriction, secretion of aldosterone from the adrenal cortex, and an intense sensation of thirst, all resulting in increased blood pressure and plasma volume. It has been recognized for some decades, however, that the brain also possesses a complete renin-angiotensin system functionally independent of the peripheral system. The central renin-angiotensin system has been shown to control secretion of the reproductive gonadotrophin hormones and also to influence learning and memory. The learning and memory aspect of the renin-angiotensin system appears to be mediated predominately by angiotensin IV, a metabolite of angiotensin II, which acts via its own receptor (insulin-regulated aminopeptidase, IRAP) which facilitates glucose uptake into cells and which catalyses the breakdown of neuromodulators such as met-enkephalin, oxytocin and vasopressin; angiotensin IV inhibits the aminopeptidase activity of IRAP (Figure 1).

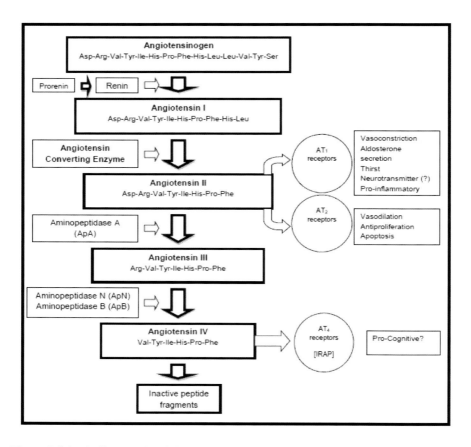

Figure 1. Metabolic cascade of the renin-angiotensin system indicating function of aminopeptidases.

We, and others, have previously shown that administration of angiotensin IV to rats and mice can improve memory acquisition, consolidation and recall (e.g., Gard et al., 2012). Furthermore it has been shown that administration of drugs known to interfere with the renin-angiotensin system, for example the anti-hypertensive ACE-inhibitors, can improve cognition in both young and old Human volunteers, probably as a consequence of elevated endogenous brain angiotensin IV (Mechaeil et al.,

2011). Acting on the hypothesis that administration of angiotensin IV may be able to reverse the deficits of learning and memory caused by prenatal alcohol exposure, we tested its effects in control mice and mice exposed to ethanol in utero at the age of 2-3 months. The pro-cognitive effect of angiotensin IV was abolished by prenatal alcohol exposure (Fidalgo et al., 2017), suggesting some alcohol-induced, long-lasting perturbation of the brain renin-angiotensin system. Subsequent research has demonstrated that angiotensin IV was unable to inhibit the aminopeptidase activity of the membrane-bound IRAP isolated from brain homogenates, suggesting some modification of the protein structure of the enzyme.

The possibility of an effect of prenatal alcohol exposure on aminopeptidase function has been followed-up in further preliminary studies of aspartyl aminopeptidase and aminopeptidases A, B, and N, all of which are involved in the synthesis of angiotensin IV from angiotensin II (see Figure 1). Studies of the membrane-bound and cytosolic components of these enzymes in brain homogenates in mice have demonstrated that prenatal alcohol exposure resulted in decreased aminopeptidase activity of IRAP in males and female offspring at two months of age, decreased brain aminopeptidase N activity in males and females, decreased brain aspartyl aminopeptidase activity in males and females, decreased brain aminopeptidase A activity in males and increased activity in females and decreased brain aminopeptidase B activity in female offspring only (Gard, 2017). The exciting aspect of these preliminary results in an animal model of FASD which has been shown to result in impaired cognition, is that the same aminopeptidases have previously been measured in human plasma and serum from patients with Alzheimer's disease, i.e., impaired cognition, and found to have decreased activity. The possibility therefore exists that decreased plasma or serum aminopeptidase activity may therefore be a correlate of decreased learning and memory. If the findings of the brain enzymes in the animal model are translated to enzyme activity, the potential for an enduring biomarker of learning impairment induced by prenatal alcohol exposure exists. Potentially more exciting, the same enzymes have also been identified and characterized in human urine, thus offering a non-invasive test of prenatal alcohol exposure.

GENETIC AND EPIGENETIC MARKERS OF FASD

More recently results from animal studies of neonatal plasma microRNA (miRNA, µRNA) have suggested that these molecules may be potential biomarkers (Mandal et al., 2018). Furthermore, DNA methylation has been identified as another potential marker of fetal alcohol exposure. That there are epigenetic changes associated with FASD is not surprising. The disease has a causation in the fetus which generally only manifests some years later in the young child. For this to occur there must be some "molecular memory" of the events occurring in the fetus. Since the majority of proteins have half-lives less than a few days, it is unlikely that changes in protein conformation or covalent modification to protein molecules would persist in the body for years. However, epigenetic changes are copied as part of the normal DNA replication process and thus inherited by daughter cells. Therefore, changes to the DNA in utero may still be present after several years.

Small, functional RNA molecules are increasingly being recognized as being functionally active biomolecules. Their roles in both healthy and diseased states are increasingly being acknowledged (Zhou and Yang, 2012). miRNA molecules are single-stranded RNAs, are typically around 21-23 nucleotides in length and are produced by the sequential cleavage of longer precursors. They are believed to function in the regulation of genes and it is estimated that at least 30% of human protein-coded genes are regulated, at least in part, by miRNA (Macfarlane and Murphy, 2010). The production of miRNA molecules is itself regulated and, therefore, the types and quantities of miRNA present in a cell will vary with environmental conditions. Although short, single-stranded RNA molecules are generally chemically unstable, they can be protected in the bloodstream by encapsulation in phospholipid vesicles or complexation with proteins (Rayner and Hennessy, 2013). Thus the presence (or absence) of specific miRNAs can be markers of disease or other adverse incidents.

In a cell culture model, miR-9, miR-21, miR-153 and miR-335 were shown to be suppressed at alcohol levels equivalent to those found in alcoholics and miR-153 was suppressed even at levels equivalent to those found in social drinkers (Sathyan et al., 2007). The consequences of reducing the amounts of these four miRNAs appear to be the induction of the cell cycle and suppression of apoptosis during neuronal development (Sathyan et al., 2007). In a sheep model, miR-9, miR-15b, miR-19b, and miR-20a were significantly altered in expression levels and plasma concentrations in both the mother and newborn lamb. Studies on human mothers demonstrated that there are similar effects on miRNA expression, albeit with a different set of miRNAs affected (miR-122*, miR-126, miR-216b, miR-221*, miR-514-5p, miR-602, miR-3119, miR-3942-5p, miR-4704-3p and miR-4743) (Gardiner et al., 2016, Balaraman et al., 2016). As such miRNAs have the potential to be used as biomarkers of dangerous levels of alcohol consumption by mothers and for identifying newborns at risk of developing FASD in the future (Balaraman et al., 2014). However, since miRNA molecules present at birth will not persist into childhood, they are unlikely to be useful for the differentiation of FASD from other conditions with similar manifestations in older children.

The methylation of DNA can affect the expression of affected genes. These covalent alterations can also be preserved through DNA replication and thus passed to daughter cells. Such epigenetic changes provide a mechanism by which developmental or environmental changes can be "remembered" through cellular lineages (Feinberg, 2018). Critically for FASD, it provides a mechanism by which the consequences of exposure to alcohol in utero can persist into childhood and beyond (Ramsay, 2010, Liyanage et al., 2017). A number of epigenetic changes have been associated with FASD (Kobor and Weinberg, 2011). Over 25 years ago, it was observed that ethanol consumption by pregnant mice reduced the methylation of DNA in the fetus. This was considered to be partly due to the inhibition of DNA methyltransferase enzymes by acetaldehyde (a product of alcohol metabolism) (Garro et al., 1991). In human males, reduced methylation at two sites (H19 and IG-DMR) was related to consumption of high levels of alcohol (Ouko et al., 2009). A similar effect on the H19 region (which controls the expression of insulin-like growth factor 2) was observed in a mouse model (Haycock and Ramsay, 2009). That this effect occurred in sperm cells suggested a possible mechanism by which excess alcohol consumption by the father might be passed on to his children. However, these particular changes do not appear to be transmitted between generations (Knezovich and Ramsay, 2012). In mouse embryos exposed to alcohol, methylation at CpG-rich promoters was reduced. However, increased methylation was observed at other sites in embryos with neural tube defects (Liu et al., 2009). In rats, methylation of the CpG dinucleotides in the proopiomelanocortin promoter was increased in neuronal cells as a consequence of alcohol consumption. This effect persisted for at least two generations in male offspring, but not in female ones (Govorko et al., 2012). However, it could be reversed by DNA methylation inhibitors (Bekdash et al., 2014). The potential role of paternal alcohol consumption in the FASD phenotype has been confirmed in mice. However, these studies suggest that inherited DNA methylation changes are not directly responsible for the phenotype and that another (as yet unidentified) epigenetic change is responsible (Chang et al., 2017). Many of the methylation changes appear to affect regions of the genome which code for non-coding RNAs, including miRNA (Laufer et al., 2013). This suggests that there is some synergism between the effects of alcohol on DNA methylation and the aberrant expression of miRNA (see above).

Recently, a number of studies have attempted to provide a global picture of epigenetic modifications which occur as a consequence of fetal alcohol exposure. One study on Canadian children identified 658 sites in the genome which are differently methylated in patients with FASD. Many of the affected genes are ones which are expressed in neuronal tissues (Portales-Casamar et al., 2016). Another study identified 259 sites and highlighted genes encoding procadherins (which assist in the proper cell-cell adhesion of neurons) among those affected (Laufer et al., 2015). These global studies suggest ways in which the methylation status of patients could be used as a biomarker of FASD (Laufer et al., 2017). There are several advantages to this approach. DNA methylation at specific sites can be relatively rapidly, cheaply and precisely determined. It is possible to determine the methylation status at numerous sites in parallel. Determination of methylation status at 161 CpG dinucleotides previously shown to be associated with FASD enabled the discrimination of FASD patients from controls. This process also differentiated the FASD patients from individuals with autism (Lussier et al., 2018). Further validation with larger sample sizes and across a variety of ethnic groups will be required before this can be developed as a robust diagnostic biomarker for FASD.

SUMMARY

Considering the studies reviewed above, it appears that six potential markers of prenatal alcohol exposure stand out as being worthy of further study: neonatal dried blood spot phosphatidylethanol, Lymphocyte β-adrenoceptors; plasma or urine F_2-isoprostanes; plasma Placental Growth Factor (PLGF), plasma or urine aminopeptidases and DNA methylation. Of these only F_2-isoprostanes and aminopeptidases have yet been associated with impaired cognition as determined in animal models, and DNA methylation has been identified in children with FASD.

REFERENCES

Abate, P., Reyes-Guzmán, A. C., Hernández-Fonseca, K. & Méndez, M. (2017). Prenatal ethanol exposure modifies locomotor activity and induces selective changes in Met-enk expression in adolescent rats. *Neuropeptides*, *62*, 45–56.

Agius, R. & Kintz, P. (2010). Guidelines for European workplace drug and alcohol testing in hair. *Drug Testing and Analysis*, *2*, 367-376.

Bakhireva, L. & Savage, D. (2011). Focus on: Biomarkers of fetal alcohol exposure and fetal alcohol effects. *Alcohol Research & Health*, *34*, 56-63.

Bakhireva, L., Leeman, L., Savich, R., Cano, S., Gutierrez, H., Savage, D. & Rayburn, W. (2014). The validity of phosphatidylethanol in dried blood spots of newborns for the identification of prenatal alcohol

exposure. *Alcoholism: Clinical and Experimental Research*, *38*, 1078-
    1085.

Balaraman, S., Lunde, E. R., Sawant, O., Cudd, T. A., Washburn, S. E. &
    Miranda, R. C. (2014). Maternal and neonatal plasma microRNA
    biomarkers for fetal alcohol exposure in an ovine model. *Alcohol Clin
    Exp Res*, *38*, 1390-400.

Balaraman, S., Schafer, J. J., Tseng, A. M., Wertelecki, W., Yevtushok, L.,
    Zymak-Zakutnya, N., Chambers, C. D. & Miranda, R. C. (2016)
    Plasma miRNA profiles in pregnant women predict infant outcomes
    following prenatal alcohol exposure. *PLoS One*, *11*, e0165081.

Banks, W. A., Wolf, K. A. & Niehoff, M. L. (2003). Effects of chronic
    ethanol on brain and serum level of methionine encephalin. *Peptides
    24*, 1935-1940.

Bearer, C., Jacobson, J., Jacobson, S., Barr, D., Croxford, J., Molteno, C.,
    Viljoen, D., Marais, A., Chiodo, L. & Cwik, A. (2003). Validation of a
    new biomarker of fetal exposure to alcohol. *The Journal of Pediatrics*,
    143, 463-469.

Bekdash, R., Zhang, C. & Sarkar, D. (2014). Fetal alcohol programming of
    hypothalamic proopiomelanocortin system by epigenetic mechanisms
    and later life vulnerability to stress. *Alcohol Clin Exp Res*, *38*, 2323-30.

Beulens, J. W. J., Van Den Berg, R., Kok, F. J., Helander, A., Vermunt, S.
    H. F. & Hendriks, H. J. (2008) Moderate alcohol consumption and
    lipoprotein-associated phospholipase A2. *Nutrition*, *Metabolism and
    Cardiovascular Diseases*, *18*, 539-544.

Brocardo, P. S., Gil-Mohapel, J., Wortman, R., Noonan, A., Mcginnis, E.,
    Patten, A. R. & Christie, B. R. (2017). The effects of ethanol exposure
    during distinct periods of brain development on oxidative stress in the
    adult rat brain. *Alcoholism: Clinical and Experimental Research*, *41*,
    26-37.

Burd, L. & Hofer, R. (2008). Biomarkers for detection of prenatal alcohol
    exposure: A critical review of fatty acid ethyl esters in meconium.
    Birth Defects Research Part A: Clinical and Molecular Teratology, *82*,
    487-493.

Cappelle, D., Neels, H., De Keukeleire, S., Fransen, E., Dom, G., Vermassen, A., Covaci, A., Crunelle, C. & Van Nuijs, A. (2017). Ethyl glucuronide in keratinous matrices as biomarker of alcohol use: A correlation study between hair and nails. *Forensic Science International, 279,* 187-191.

Carstens, M. E., Engelbrecht, A. H., Russell, V. A., Aalbers, C., Gagiano, C. A., Chalton, D. O. & Taljaard, J. J. (1987). Beta-adrenoceptors on lymphocytes of patients with major depressive disorder. *Psychiatry Res., 20,* 239–48.

Cederbaum, A. I. (2012). Alcohol metabolism. *Clin. Liver Dis., 16,* 2012, 667-685.

Chan, D., Knie, B. & Koren, G. (2004). Placental handling of fatty acid ethyl esters: perfusion and subcellular studies. *Journal of Pharmacology and Experimental Therapeutics, 310,* 75-82.

Chang, R. C., Skiles, W. M., Chronister, S. S., Wang, H., Sutton, G. I., Bedi, Y. S., Snyder, M., Long, C. R. & Golding, M. C. (2017) DNA methylation-independent growth restriction and altered developmental programming in a mouse model of preconception male alcohol exposure. *Epigenetics, 12,* 841-853.

Crunelle, C., Verbeek, J., Dom, G., Covaci, A., Yegles, M., Michielsen, P., De Doncker, M., Nevens, F., Cappelle, D., Van Nuijs, A. & Neels, H. (2016). Hair ethyl glucuronide and serum carbohydrate deficient transferrin for the assessment of relapse in alcohol-dependent patients. *Clinical Biochemistry, 49,* 554-559.

De Carvalho, J., Piva, S., Hausen, B., Bochi, G., Kaefer, M., Coelho, A., Duarte, M. & Moresco, R. (2011). Assessment of urinary γ-glutamyltransferase and alkaline phosphatase for diagnosis of diabetic nephropathy. *Clinica Chimica Acta, 412,* 1407-1411.

Dresen, S., Weinmann, W. & Wurst, F. (2004). Forensic confirmatory analysis of ethyl sulfate—A new marker for alcohol consumption—by liquid-chromatography/electrospray ionization/tandem mass spectrometry. *Journal of the American Society for Mass Spectrometry, 15,* 1644-1648.

Duman, R. S., Heninger, G. R. & Nestler, E. J. (1997). A molecular and cellular theory of depression. *Arch. Gen. Psychiatr.*, *54*, 597-606.

Feinberg, A. P. (2018). The key role of epigenetics in human disease prevention and mitigation. *N Engl J Med*, *378*, 1323-1334.

Fidalgo, S., Skipper, C., Takyi, A., Mciver, A., Tsiligkaridis, T., Quadir, A. & Gard, P. R. (2017). Low-dose chronic prenatal alcohol exposure abolishes the pro-cognitive effects of Angiotensin IV. *Behavioural Brain Research*, *329*, 140-147.

Fontaine, C. J., Pattena, A. R., Sickmann, H. M., Helfera, J. L., Brian, R. & Christie, B. R. (2016). Effects of pre-natal alcohol exposure on hippocampal synaptic plasticity: Sex, age and methodological considerations. *Neuroscience and Biobehavioral Reviews*, *64*, 12–34.

Franzini, M., Fornaciari, I., Vico, T., Moncini, M., Cellesi, V., Meini, M., Emdin, M. & Paolicchi, A. (2013). High-sensitivity gamma-glutamyltransferase fraction pattern in alcohol addicts and abstainers. *Drug and Alcohol Dependence*, *127*, 239-242.

Fukuda, K., Baba, A., Nakamura, Y., Kuchii, M., Nishio, I. & Masuyama, Y. (1985) Decreased concentrations of lymphocyte and platelet β-adrenoceptors in spontaneously hypertensive rats. *Japanese Heart Journal*, *26*, 662.

Gard, P. R., Naylor, C., Ali, S. & Partington, C. (2012). Blockade of pro-cognitive effects of angiotensin IV and physostigmine in mice by oxytocin antagonism. *Eur. J. Pharmacol.*, *683*, 155-160.

Gard, P. R. (2017). Serum aminopeptidase activity as a potential persistent marker of prenatal alcohol exposure. *Presented to the 7th International Conference on Fetal Alcohol Spectrum Disorder*, Vancouver, Canada.

Gardiner, A. S., Gutierrez, H. L., Luo, L., Davies, S., Savage, D. D., Bakhireva, L. N. & Perrone-Bizzozero, N. I. (2016). Alcohol use during pregnancy is associated with specific alterations in microrna levels in maternal serum. *Alcohol Clin Exp Res*, *40*, 826-37.

Garro, A. J., Mcbeth, D. L., Lima, V. & Lieber, C. S. (1991). Ethanol consumption inhibits fetal DNA methylation in mice: implications for the fetal alcohol syndrome. *Alcohol Clin Exp Res*, *15*, 395-8.

Golding, B. J., Overall, A. D. J., Brown, G. & Gard, P. R. (2010). Strain differences in the effects of angiotensin IV on mouse cognition. *Eur. J. Pharmacol.*, *641*, 154-159.

Golka, K., Sondermann, R., Reich, S. & Wiese, A. (2004). Carbohydrate-deficient transferrin (CDT) as a biomarker in persons suspected of alcohol abuse. *Toxicology Letters*, *151*, 235-241.

Govorko, D., Bekdash, R. A., Zhang, C. & Sarkar, D. K. (2012). Male germline transmits fetal alcohol adverse effect on hypothalamic proopiomelanocortin gene across generations. *Biol Psychiatry*, *72*, 378-88.

Gottesfeld, Z., Morgan, B., Perzpolo, J. R. (1990). Prenatal alcohol exposure alters the development of sympathetic synaptic components and of nerve growth-factor receptor expression selectivity in lymphoid organs. *J. Neurosci. Res*, *26*, 308-316.

Halmesmaki, E., Roine, R. & Salaspuro, M. (1992). Gamma glutarayl-transferase, aspartate and alamine aminotransferases and their ratio, mean cell volume and urinary dolichol in pregnant alcohol abusers. *International Journal of Gynecology & Obstetrics*, *40*, 87-87.

Haycock, P. C. & Ramsay, M. (2009). Exposure of mouse embryos to ethanol during preimplantation development: effect on DNA methylation in the h19 imprinting control region. *Biol Reprod*, *81*, 618-27.

Himes, S., Dukes, K., Tripp, T., Petersen, J., Raffo, C., Burd, L., Odendaal, H., Elliott, A., Hereld, D., Signore, C., Willinger, M. & Huestis, M. (2015). Clinical sensitivity and specificity of meconium fatty acid ethyl ester, ethyl glucuronide, and ethyl sulfate for detecting maternal drinking during pregnancy. *Clinical Chemistry*, *61*, 523-532.

Howlett, H., Abernethy, S., Brown, N., Rankin, J. & Gray, W. (2017). How strong is the evidence for using blood biomarkers alone to screen for alcohol consumption during pregnancy? A systematic review. *European Journal of Obstetrics & Gynecology and Reproductive Biology*, *213*, 45-52.

Jacobson, J., Jacobson, S., Sokol, R. & Ager, J. (1998). Relation of maternal age and pattern of pregnancy drinking to functionally significant cognitive deficit in infancy. *Alcoholism: Clinical & Experimental Research, 22*, 345-351.

Joya, X., Friguls, B., Ortigosa, S., Papaseit, E., Martínez, S., Manich, A., Garcia-Algar, O., Pacifici, R., Vall, O. & Pichini, S. (2012). Determination of maternal-fetal biomarkers of prenatal exposure to ethanol: A review. *Journal of Pharmaceutical and Biomedical Analysis, 69*, 209-222.

Joya, X., Marchei, E., Salat-Batlle, J., García-Algar, O., Calvaresi, V., Pacifici, R. & Pichini, S. (2016). Fetal exposure to ethanol: relationship between ethyl glucuronide in maternal hair during pregnancy and ethyl glucuronide in neonatal meconium. *Clinical Chemistry and Laboratory Medicine, 54*, 427-435.

Kenan, N., Larsson, A., Axelsson, O. & Helander, A. (2011). Changes in transferrin glycosylation during pregnancy may lead to false-positive carbohydrate-deficient transferrin (CDT) results in testing for riskful alcohol consumption. *Clinica Chimica Acta, 412*, 129-133.

Kissack, J., Bishop, J. & Roper, A. (2008). Ethylglucuronide as a biomarker for ethanol detection. *Pharmacotherapy, 28*, 769-781.

Kwak, H., Han, J., Ahn, H., Kim, M., Ryu, H., Kim, M., Chung, H., Cho, D., Shin, C., Velazquez-Armenta, E. & Nava-Ocampo, A. (2012). Blood levels of phosphatidylethanol in pregnant women reporting positive alcohol ingestion, measured by an improved LC-MS/MS analytical method. *Clinical Toxicology, 50*, 886-891.

Knezovich, J. G. & Ramsay, M. (2012). The effect of preconception paternal alcohol exposure on epigenetic remodeling of the H19 and Rasgrf1 imprinting control regions in mouse offspring. *Front Genet, 3*, article 10.

Kobor, M. S. & Weinberg, J. (2011). Focus on: epigenetics and fetal alcohol spectrum disorders. *Alcohol Res Health, 34*, 29-37.

Koren, G., Chan, D., Klein, J. & Karaskov, T. (2002). Estimation of fetal exposure to drugs of abuse, environmental tobacco smoke, and ethanol. *Therapeutic Drug Monitoring, 24*, 23-25.

Kwong, T. & Ryan, R. (1997). Detection of intrauterine illicit drug exposure by newborn drug testing. *Clinical Chemistry, 43*, 235-242.

Lange, S., Shield, K., Koren, G., Rehm, J. & Popova, S. (2014). A comparison of the prevalence of prenatal alcohol exposure obtained via maternal self-reports versus meconium testing: a systematic literature review and meta-analysis. *BMC Pregnancy and Childbirth*, *14*, article 127.

Laske, A., Stransky, E., Leyle, T., Eschweiler, G. W., Maetzler, W., Wittorfe, A., Soekadar, S., Richartz, E., Koehler, N., Bartels, M., Buchkremer, G. & Schott, K. (2007). BDNF serum and CSF concentrations in Alzheimer's disease, normal pressure hydrocephalus and healthy controls. *J. Psych. Res.*, *41*, 387–394.

Laufer, B. I., Chater-Diehl, E. J., Kapalanga, J. & Singh, S. M. (2017). Long-term alterations to DNA methylation as a biomarker of prenatal alcohol exposure: From mouse models to human children with fetal alcohol spectrum disorders. *Alcohol*, *60*, 67-75.

Laufer, B. I., Kapalanga, J., Castellani, C. A., Diehl, E. J., Yan, L. & Singh, S. M. (2015). Associative DNA methylation changes in children with prenatal alcohol exposure. *Epigenomics*, *7*, 1259-74.

Laufer, B. I., Mantha, K., Kleiber, M. L., Diehl, E. J., Addison, S. M. & Singh, S. M. (2013). Long-lasting alterations to DNA methylation and ncRNAs could underlie the effects of fetal alcohol exposure in mice. *Dis Model Mech*, *6*, 977-92.

Lecuyer, M., Laquerriere, A., Bekri, S., Lesueur, C., Ramdani, Y., Jegou, S., et al. (2017). PLGF, a placental marker of fetal brain defects after in utero alcohol exposure. *Acta Neuropathol. Commun.*, *5*.

Lee, S. J., Baek, J. H. & Kim, Y. H. (2009). Brain-derived neurotrophic factor is associated with cognitive impairment in elderly Korean individuals. *Clin. Psychopharmacol. Neurosci.*, *13*, 283-287.

Lee, D., Ha, M., Kim, J., Gross, M. & Jacobs, D. (2002). Gamma-glutamyltransferase, alcohol, and blood pressure: a four year follow-up study. *Annals of Epidemiology*, *12*(2), pp. 90-96.

Lee, S., Choi, E., Han, K., Cha, M. & Oh, S. (2017). Association between γ-glutamyltransferase level and incidence of atrial fibrillation: A nationwide population-based study. *International Journal of Cardiology*, *245*, 149-155.

Littner, Y. & Bearer, C. (2007). Detection of alcohol consumption during pregnancy—Current and future biomarkers. *Neuroscience & Biobehavioral Reviews*, *31*, 261-269.

Liu, Y., Balaraman, Y., Wang, G., nephew, K. P. & Zhou, F. C. (2009) Alcohol exposure alters DNA methylation profiles in mouse embryos at early neurulation. *Epigenetics*, *4*, 500-11.

Liu, X., Zhang, J., Sun, D., Fan, Y., Zhou, H. & Fu, B. (2014). Effects of fluoxetine on brain-derived neurotrophic factor serum concentration and cognition in patients with vascular dementia. *Clin. Invest. in Aging*, *9*, 411-418.

Liyanage, V. R., Curtis, K., Zachariah, R. M., Chudley, A. E. & Rastegar, M. (2017) Overview of the genetic basis and epigenetic mechanisms that contribute to FASD pathobiology. *Curr Top Med Chem*, *17*, 808-828.

Lussier, A. A., Morin, A. M., Macisaac, J. L., Salmon, J., Weinberg, J., Reynolds, J. N., Pavlidis, P., Chudley, A. E. & Kobor, M. S. (2018). DNA methylation as a predictor of fetal alcohol spectrum disorder. *Clin Epigenetics*, *10*, article 5.

Macfarlane, L. A. & Murphy, P. R. (2010). MicroRNA: Biogenesis, function and role in cancer. *Curr Genomics*, *11*, 537-61.

Mandal, C., Halder, D., Jung, K. H. & Chai, Y. G. (2018). Maternal alcohol consumption and altered miRNAs in the developing fetus: Context and future perspectives. *J Appl Toxicol*, *38*, 100-107.

Mechaeil, R., Lewis, M., Grice, J., Gard, P. R., Jackson, A. & Rusted, J. (2011). Angiotensin receptor antagonists as potential cognitive enhancing agents. *Psychopharmacol.*, *217*, 51-60.

Milne, G. L.., Qi, D., Roberts, L. & Jackson, I. I. (2015). The isoprostanes-25 years later. *Biochim. Biophys. Acta. Molecular Cell Biology of Lipids.*, *1851*, 433-445.

Moore, C., Jones, J., Lewis, D. & Buchi, K. (2003). Prevalence of fatty acid ethyl esters in meconium specimens. *Clinical Chemistry*, *49*, 133-136.

Morini, L., Marchei, E., Vagnarelli, F., Garcia Algar, O., Groppi, A., Mastrobattista, L. & Pichini, S. (2010). Ethyl glucuronide and ethyl sulfate in meconium and hair-potential biomarkers of intrauterine exposure to ethanol. *Forensic Science International, 196*, 74-77.

Morini, L., Politi, L. & Polettini, A. (2009). Ethyl glucuronide in hair. A sensitive and specific marker of chronic heavy drinking. *Addiction, 104*, 915-920.

Naegelin, Y., Dingsdale, H., Sauberli, K., Schedelin, S., Kappos, L. & Barde, Y. A. (In Press). *Measuring and Validating the Levels of Brain-Derived Neurotrophic Factor in Human Serum.* eNeuro.

Ostrea, E., Hernandez, J., Bielawski, D., Kan, J., Leonardo, G., Abela, M., Church, M., Hannigan, J., Janisse, J., Ager, J. & Sokol, R. (2006). Fatty acid ethyl esters in meconium: are they biomarkers of fetal alcohol exposure and effect? *Alcoholism: Clinical and Experimental Research, 30*, 1152-1159.

Ouko, L. A., Shantikumar, K., Knezovich, J., haycock, P., Schnugh, D. J. & Ramsay, M. (2009) Effect of alcohol consumption on CpG methylation in the differentially methylated regions of H19 and IG-DMR in male gametes: implications for fetal alcohol spectrum disorders. *Alcohol Clin Exp Res, 33*, 1615-27.

Petrelli, B., Weinberg, J., HICKS, G. G. (in press). Effects of prenatal exposure (PAE): Insights into FASD using PAE mouse models. *Biochem. Cell. Biol.*

Politi, L., Morini, L., Leone, F. & Polettini, A. (2006). Ethyl glucuronide in hair: is it a reliable marker of chronic high levels of alcohol consumption? *Addiction, 101*, 1408-1412.

Portales-Casamar, E., Lussier, A. A., Jones, M. J., Macisaac, J. L., Edgar, R. D., Mah, S. M., Barhdadi, A., Provost, S., Lemieux-Perreault, L. P., Cynader, M. S., Chudley, A. E., Dube, M. P., Reynolds, J. N., Pavlidis, P. & Kobor, M. S. (2016). DNA methylation signature of human fetal alcohol spectrum disorder. *Epigenetics Chromatin, 9*, article 25.

Pragst, F., Auwaerter, V., Sporkert, F. & Spiegel, K. (2001). Analysis of fatty acid ethyl esters in hair as possible markers of chronically elevated alcohol consumption by headspace solid-phase micro-extraction (HS-SPME) and gas chromatography-mass spectrometry (GC-MS). *Forensic Science International, 121*, 76-88.

Quinn, M. E., Grant, K. E. & Adam, E. K. (2018). Negative cognitive style and cortisol recovery accentuate the relationship between life stress and depressive symptoms. *Stress-The International Journal on the Biology of Stress.*, *21*, 119-127.

Raineki, C., Bodnar, T. S., Holman, P. J., Baglot, S. L., Lan, N. & Weinberg, J. (2017). Effects of early-life adversity on immune function are mediated by prenatal environment: Role of prenatal alcohol exposure. *Brain, Behavior, and Immunity*, *66*, 210–220.

Ramsay, M. (2010). Genetic and epigenetic insights into fetal alcohol spectrum disorders. *Genome Med*, *2*, article 27.

Rayner, K. J. & Hennessy, E. J. (2013). Extracellular communication via microRNA: lipid particles have a new message. *J Lipid Res*, *54*, 1174-81.

Sathyan, P., Golden, H. B. & Miranda, R. C. (2007). Competing interactions between micro-RNAs determine neural progenitor survival and proliferation after ethanol exposure: evidence from an ex vivo model of the fetal cerebral cortical neuroepithelium. *J Neurosci*, *27*, 8546-57.

Schambra, U. B., Lewis, C. N. & Harrison, T. A. (2017). Deficits in spatial learning and memory in adult mice following acute, low or moderate levels of prenatal ethanol exposure during gastrulation or neurulation. *Neurotoxicol. Teratol.*, *62*, 42-54.

Seebacher, V., Polterauer, S., Grimm, C., Rahhal, J., Hofstetter, G., Bauer, E., Husslein, H., Leipold, H., Marth, C., Reinthaller, A. & Concin, N. (2012). Prognostic significance of gamma-glutamyltransferase in patients with endometrial cancer: a multi-centre trial. *British Journal of Cancer*, *106*, 1551-1555.

Sen, S., Duman, R. & Sanacora, G. (2008). Serum brain-derived neurotrophic factor, depression, and antidepressant medications: meta-analyes and implications. *Biol. Psychiatr*, *64*, 527-532.

Subedi, L., Huang, H., Pant, A., Westgate, P. M., Bada, H. S., Bauer, J. A., Giannone, P. J. & Sithisarn, T. (2017). Plasma Brain-Derived neurotrophic Factor levels in newborn infants with neonatal abstinence syndrome. *Frontiers in Pediatric*, *5*, article 238.

Streissguth, A., Sampson, P., Olson, H., Bookstein, F., Barr, H., Scott, M., Feldman, J. & Mirsky, A. (1994). Maternal Drinking During Pregnancy: Attention and Short-Term Memory in 14-Year-Old Offspring-A Longitudinal Prospective Study. *Alcoholism: Clinical and Experimental Research, 18,* 202-218.

Taracha, E., Habrat, B., Lehner, M., Wislowska, A., Woronowicz, B., Bogulas, M., Charewicz, J., Markuszewski, C. & Plaźnik, A. (2004). Alanine Aminopeptidase Activity in Urine: A New Marker of Chronic Alcohol Abuse? *Alcoholism: Clinical and Experimental Research, 28,* 729-735.

Terasaki, L. S. & Schwarz, J. M. (2017). Impact of Prenatal and Subsequent Adult Alcohol Exposure on Pro-Inflammatory Cytokine Expression in Brain Regions Necessary for Simple Recognition Memory. *Brain Sci., 7,* article 125.

Varga, A., Hansson, P., Johnson, G. & Alling, C. (2000). Normalization rate and cellular localization of phosphatidylethanol in whole blood from chronic alcoholics. *Clinica Chimica Acta, 299,* 141-150.

Viel, G., Boscolo-Berto, R., Cecchetto, G., Fais, P., Nalesso, A. & Ferrara, S. (2012). Phosphatidylethanol in Blood as a Marker of Chronic Alcohol Use: A Systematic Review and Meta-Analysis. *International Journal of Molecular Sciences, 13,* 14788-14812.

Wolff, K. & Marshall, E. (2006). Biological markers of alcohol use. *Psychiatry, 5,* 437-438.

Xia, L. P., Shen, L., Kou, H., Zhang, B. J., Zhang, L., Wu, Y., Li, X. J., Xiong, J., Yu, Y. & Wang, H. (2014). Prenatal ethanol exposure enhances the susceptibility to metabolic syndrome in offspring rats by HPA axis-associated neuroendocrinemetabolic programming. *Toxicology Letters, 226,* 98–105.

Zhou, X. & Yang, P. C. (2012) MicroRNA: a small molecule with a big biological impact. *MicroRNA, 1,* article 1.

In: Fetal Alcohol Syndrome
Editor: Doug Knight

ISBN: 978-1-53614-602-8
© 2018 Nova Science Publishers, Inc.

Chapter 3

NEURON-MICROGLIA INTERACTIONS IN FETAL ALCOHOL SPECTRUM DISORDERS

Nadka I. Boyadjieva*, MD, PhD, DSci,
Miroslava G. Varadinova, MD, PhD,
Ivailo A. Bogomilov, MD,
Georgi A. Bogdanov MD, PhD,
Rumen P. Nikolov MD, PhD
and Rositza D. Metodieva
Department of Pharmacology and Toxicology, Medical Faculty,
Medical University, Sofia, Bulgaria

ABSTRACT

Fetal alcohol spectrum disorder (FASD) is a result of maternal consumption of alcohol during pregnancy. This chapter summarizes data from investigations of the effects of alcohol on neuron-microglia interactions. It is based on recent findings in models of FASD which demonstrate that alcohol causes loss of both neurons and microglia in the

---

* Corresponding Author Email: nadkaboyadjieva@gmail.com.

developing brain. The chapter presents structural and functional characteristics of neuron-microglia interactions as well as the effects of alcohol on various cytokines which play roles in the mechanisms of those interactions. The consequences of glial nitric oxide synthase activity in the apoptotic effects of ethanol on developing neurons are also illustrated. The key factors regulated by the microglia-specific signal transducer and activator of transcription 3 in neuron–microglia interactions are analyzed. Overall, the chapter summarizes the long-term effects of fetal alcohol exposure on neuronal plasticity.

NEURON-MICROGLIA INTERACTIONS

Glia consists of non-neuronal cells in the central and in the peripheral nervous system. They play a role in maintaining homeostasis, formation of myelin, and protecting the neurons [1]. The most common glial cells in the central nervous system (CNS) are oligodendrocytes, astrocytes, ependymal cells, and microglia. Glial cells have primarily supportive role for the neurons but they also regulate the internal environment of the brain the neurotransmission and the synaptic plasticity play a role in neuro-transmission and synaptic connections [2]. During early embryogenesis, glial cells direct the migration of neurons and produce molecules that modify neurogenesis. The most numerous macroglial cells in the CNS are the astrocytes, which have a key role in forming the blood-brain barrier and are responsible for the regulation of the environment surrounding the neurons as well. The second largest group of glial cells in the brain is microglia. Microglia are the primary cells to mediate immune response in the CNS and participate in the immune regulation, cytotoxic response and injury resolution [3]. Microglial cells are found in all regions of the brain and are mainly involved in the inflammation and neurodegeneration processes associated with brain damages [4].

The classical M1-phenotype of microglia is associated with cytotoxicity and inflammatory responses, while the alternative M2-phenotype is regarded as being beneficial. Minocycline selectively inhibits M1 polarization of microglia and supports the data for inflammatory role of M1-type activation of microglial cells [5]. The classification of microglial activation phenotypes on neurodegeneration and regeneration in Alzheimer's disease brain also confirm the data about the dual role of microglia in the CNS [6]. Microglia are known to secrete neurotrophins and protective cytokines to promote neuronal development and survival. However, upon CNS insult or injury, microglia can acquire complex phenotypes in order to participate in the cytotoxic response, immune regulation, and injury effects. It has been shown that chronic alcohol consumption activates microglia to a M1-phenotype and promotes inflammatory responses [4]. Activation of microglia to the M1-phenotype is crucial during the developmental period, since it may lead to fetal ethanol neurotoxicity and developmental disorders [7].

Recently, it has been shown that microglial activity is tightly controlled by communication between neurons and microglia both under healthy and pathological conditions. Under stress, neurons may release immunomodulatory factors and signaling molecules including neuro-transmitters, which may recruit microglia proximally to the affected neurons and induce activation of microglia [8, 9, 10, 11]. Mechanisms for the bi-directional communication between activated microglia and neurons may include numerous types of neurotransmitter receptors which are present on microglia [12]. Eyo & Wu (2013) reported for a bidirectional neuron-microglia communication in the healthy brain as well as in injured developing brain [8]. The participation of various receptors in neuron-microglia interactions are a subject of lots of studies. The role of cholinergic and noradrenergic systems in neuron-microglia interaction in inflammatory and degenerative diseases is suggested [9, 10]. Neuro-transmitter receptors on microglia are recognized [12]. The presence of mu-opioid receptors (MOR) in microglia has been previously demonstrated by immunocytochemistry, Western blot, and PCR detections in the CNS [13]. Some studies detected delta-opioid receptor (DOR) proteins by immunocytochemistry and RT-PCR in primary cultures of forebrain microglial cells [14], but others failed to detect DOR proteins by a similar technique in primary microglial cultures from the cortical area of the brain [15].

FETAL ALCOHOL EXPOSURE
AND NEURON-MICROGLIA INTERACTIONS

Alcohol exposure has many detrimental effects on the developing brain and has been known to cause FASD. Wilhelm & Guizzetti (2016) analyzed the role of microglia in FASD (16). Studies in fetal and neonatal animal models show that ethanol may stimulate neuron cell death, at least in part, through stimulation of neuroinflammatory and neurodegenerative processes in the CNS. Alcohol exposure affects the viability of neurons following neonatal alcohol exposure, and peroxisome proliferator-activated receptor-γ (PPAR-γ) agonists limit this ethanol-induced cell loss [17]. Repeated alcohol exposure during the developmental period may also lead to long-term sensitization of microglia which results in persistent pro-inflammatory signaling in the brain following damage [18].

Maternal ethanol consumption affects normal fetal brain growth and reduces neuronal density in various brain regions. Numerous mechanisms demonstrate ethanol toxicity on the developing brain [19, 20, 21, 22, 23]. Apoptosis plays an important role in fetal alcohol disorders. Our published data documented for the first time that cyclic adenosine monophosphate (cAMP) and ethanol interacted to control apoptosis and differentiation in hypothalamic beta-endorphin neurons [20]. We also reported the role of microglia in the ethanol pro-apoptotic action on hypothalamic neuronal cells in primary cultures [24]. Microglial activation and inflammatory molecules expression as a result of ethanol treatment have been well studied during brain development [18, 25, 26]. It has been shown that high doses of ethanol during the developmental period activate microglia to a pro-inflammatory stage. Studies also demonstrated that the prenatal ethanol exposure may increase the expression of neuroinflammatory cytokines and chemokines in diverse regions of the brain.

Prenatal ethanol produces alteration of the body's clock regulatory mechanisms within the suprachiasmatic nucleus of the hypothalamus [27]. Many of the hypothalamic functional defects in prenatal ethanol-exposed animals are related to a loss of neuronal cell population [20; 28; 29].

Prenatal ethanol has been shown to induce morphological and functional abnormalities of various neuronal populations including those producing β-endorphin [29], luteinizing hormone-releasing hormone [30], corticotropin-releasing hormone [31], alpha-melanocyte-stimulating hormone, neuropeptide Y, galanin [32], orexin 1 [33], vasoactive intestinal peptide [34], etc. Our previous studies have demonstrated that ethanol treatment increases the release of various cytokines such as TNF-α, IL-1β, IL-6 from the microglial cells and that TNF-α causes apoptotic cell death of developing hypothalamic neurons *in vitro* [35].

Recently, oxidative stress has been proposed as a mechanism of ethanol teratogenicity [36]. Ramachandran et al. (2003), reported that ethanol-induced oxidative stress preceded mitochondrially-mediated apoptotic death of cultured fetal cortical neurons [37]. After ethanol administration formation of reactive oxygen species (ROS) occurs intracellularly in various tissues of rodent species [38]. Experimental data have indicated that microglia are a source of ROS in the brain [39; 40]. The production of ROS by the microglial cells is a part of the immune defense in the brain. A limited number of studies have focused on the role of ROS generated from microglia in the process of apoptotic neuronal death [41, 42]. However, the role of ROS produced by ethanol-treated microglia in the apoptosis of developing hypothalamic neurons is not well studied. For the first time, we have determined that ethanol-treated microglial cell cultures generate ROS and increase the apoptotic cell death of fetal hypothalamic neurons [43]. Our results demonstrated that treatment with ethanol increased oxidative stress in neuronal cultures, detected by higher cellular levels of oxidants and lower levels of antioxidants and antioxidative enzymes, as well as, increased apoptotic death. In addition, the effects of ethanol on oxidative stress and cell death were enhanced in the presence of microglia. Moreover, antioxidative agents protected developing hypothalamic neurons from the oxidative stress and the cellular apoptosis, caused by ethanol or ethanol-treated microglial culture medium. ROS have been implicated in oxidative stress induction and as a factor in enhanced apoptosis in fetal brains exposed to ethanol in utero [44]. Chao et al. (1992) demonstrated that activated microglia mediated neuronal cell injury via a nitric oxide mechanism [39].

Ethanol decreased the levels of the powerful endogenous antioxidant glutathione (GSH) [45] and the activity of the enzyme glutathione peroxidase (GSH-Px) in neurons. The role of GSH in ethanol-related toxicity is well documented in the liver [46]. Maffi et al. (2008) suggest that the GSH content is an important predictor of the neuronal sensitivity to ethanol-mediated oxidative stress and subsequent cell death [47]. The view that the GSH content is important for prevention of prenatal ethanol neurotoxicity is supported from various studies which document that normalizing or enhancing GSH levels in cultured cerebral cortical neurons can prevent ethanol-mediated oxidative stress and decrease the apoptotic cell death [37, 48]. In agreement with other studies our data demonstrated that ethanol decreased GSH levels and GSH-Px activity and also increased the apoptosis of developing hypothalamic cells.

Microglial cells are a source of various substances, part of which are well-recognized with their toxicity on neurons. We have previously reported that ethanol-treated cultured microglia produce various cytokines as TNF-α, IL-ß MIP-1, MIP-2 (Boyadjieva and Sarkar, 2010). The cytokine production is essential for the polarization of microglia into what has been termed as classically activated, M1 state [6]. As mentioned above, microglial cells are a powerful source of reactive oxygen and nitrogen species as well [49]. Taken together, the data from studies on fetal alcohol effects provide evidence that microglial cell-derived substances enhance the effects of ethanol on inflammation and apoptosis, via disruption of the oxidant/antioxidant balance in developing hypothalamic neurons. Cohen-Kerem & Koren (2003) analyzed various data from experimental studies and their implications to humans and verified the protective role of antioxidants against ethanol teratogenicity [36]. Whether or not microglia induces oxidative stress and apoptosis in neurons via microglia-derived proinflammatory cytokines and/or free radicals remains to be fully elucidated. Now, it is well established that the activation of glial cells is a critical event in many neuroinflammatory processes [49, 50]. Proinflammatory cytokines and free radicals may cause both neuroinflammation and neurodegeneration and act as neurotoxic factors activated by ethanol [24, 51, 52, 53].

Another direction of our investigation has focused on the detrimental effects of fetal alcohol exposure on hypothalamic proopiomelanocortin (POMC) neurons, which are known to produce opioid peptides [13]. We have determined that fetal alcohol exposure increases POMC neuronal death [54]. Opioid receptors on microglia may be potential target molecules for fetal alcohol toxicity. Furthermore, various studies report abnormalities in the feedback regulation of stress axis function during a stress challenge of neonates after fetal alcohol exposure [55, 56, 57, 58]. Both types of opioid receptors MOR and DOR are known to be involved in the communication between POMC neurons and microglia during ethanol toxicity. Using *in vivo* model of neonatal alcohol feeding rat and *in vitro* model of primary cultures of rat hypothalamic microglia and neural stem cell-derived POMC cells, we evaluated the role of MOR and DOR in ethanol activation of microglia to promote apoptotic action on POMC neurons. Our studies demonstrated that alcohol neurotoxic action on POMC neurons resulted into dysregulated expression and action of MOR and DOR to promote MOR-activated neuroinflammatory signaling and to reduce DOR-regulated anti-inflammatory signaling in microglia [59]. For the first time we showed that ethanol and a MOR agonist increased the secretion of pro-inflammatory cytokines but decreased the secretion of anti-inflammatory cytokines, while a DOR agonist decreased the secretion of pro-inflammatory cytokines but increased the secretion of anti-inflammatory cytokines from the microglia. In addition, ethanol's apoptotic action on POMC neurons was prevented by DOR-activated production of IL-4 and IL-13. Taken together, our data suggest that opioid receptors MOR and DOR differentially respond to the ethanol challenge and differentially control the production of inflammatory and anti-inflammatory cytokines from microglia to control POMC neuronal apoptosis. The role of activated microglia in ethanol-induced fetal and neonatal toxicity as well as the protective effect of a DOR agonist in neuronal apoptosis may present a future approach for understanding fetal alcohol spectrum diseases.

REFERENCES

[1]   Jessen K, Mirsky R. (1980). Glial cells in the enteric nervous system contain glial fibrillary acidic protein. *Nature*, 286 (5774):736-737.

[2]   Schafer D, Stevens B. (2015). Microglia Function in Central Nervous System Development and Plasticity. *Cold Spring Harb Perspect Biol.* 7(10):a020545.

[3]   Bilbo S, Schwarz J. (2012). The immune system and developmental programming of brain and behavior. *Front Neuroendocrinol.*, 33:267–286.

[4]   Sierra A, Tremblay M, Wake H. (2014). Never-resting microglia: physiological roles in the healthy brain and pathological implications. *Front. Cell. Neurosci.* 8:240.

[5]   Chhor V, Le Charpentier T, Lebon S, Oré M, Celador I, Josserand J, et al. (2013). Characterization of phenotype markers and neuro-notoxic potential of polarised primary microglia *in vitro*. *Brain Behav Immun.*, 32:70–85.

[6]   Varnum M, Ikezu T. (2012). The classification of microglial activation phenotypes on neurodegeneration and regeneration in Alzheimer's disease brain. *Arch Immunol Ther Exp* (Warsz), 60:251–266.

[7]   Bell-Temin H, Zhang P, Chaput D, King M, You M, Liu B, Stevens S., Jr. Quantitative proteomic characterization of ethanol-responsive pathways in rat microglial cells. *J Proteome Res.* 2013; 12:2067–2077.

[8]   Eyo U, Wu L. (2013). Bidirectional microglia-neuron communication in the healthy brain. *Neural Plasticity*, 456857.

[9]   Carnevale D, De Simone R, Minghetti L. (2007). Microglia-neuron interaction in inflammatory and degenerative diseases: role of cholinergic and noradrenergic systems. *CNS Neurol Disord Drug Targets.*, 6 (6):388–397.

[10] Sheridan G, Murphy K. (2013). Neuron—glia crosstalk in health and disease: fractalkine and CX3CR1 take centre stage. *Open Biol.*, 3:130181.

[11] Wohleb E, Franklin T, Iwata M, Duman R. (2016). Integrating neuroimmune systems in the neurobiology of depression. *Nat Rev Neurosci.*, 17:497–11.

[12] Liu H, Leak R, Hu X. (2016). Neurotransmitter receptors on microglia. *Stroke Vasc Neurol.*, 1.

[13] Hadley M, Haskell-Luevano C. (1999). The proopiomelanocortin system. *Ann N Y Acad Sci.*, 885:1–21.

[14] Turchan-Cholewo J, Dimayuga F, Ding Q, Keller J, Hauser K, Knapp P, et al. (2008). Cell-specific actions of HIV-Tat and morphine on opioid receptor expression in glia. *J Neurosci Res.*, 86:2100–2110.

[15] Mika J, Popiolek-Barczyk K, Rojewska E, Makuch W, Starowicz K, Przewlocka B. (2014). Delta-opioid receptor analgesia is independent of microglial activation in a rat model of neuropathic pain. *PLoS One*, 9.

[16] Wilhelm C, Guizzetti M. (2016). Fetal alcohol spectrum disorders: an overview from the glia perspective. *Front Integr Neurosci.*, 9:65.

[17] Kane C, Phelan K, Han L, Smith R, Xie J, Douglas J, et al. (2011). Protection of neurons and microglia against ethanol in a mouse model of fetal alcohol spectrum disorders by peroxisome proliferator-activated receptor-γ agonists. *Brain Behav Immun.*, 1 (25): S137–S145.

[18] Chastain L, Sarkar D. (2014). Role of microglia in regulation of ethanol neurotoxic action. *Int Rev Neurobiol.*, 118:81–03.

[19] Chen W, Maier S, Parnell S, West J. (2003). Alcohol and the developing brain: neuroanatomical studies. *Alcohol Res Health.*, 27:174–180.

[20] De A, Boyadjieva N, Pastorcic M, Reddy B, Sarkar D. (1994). Cyclic AMP and ethanol interact to control apoptosis and differentiation in hypothalamic beta-endorphin neurons. *J Biol Chem.*, 269:26697–26705.

[21] Goodlett C, Thomas J, West J. (1991). Long-term deficits in cerebellar growth and rotarod performance of rats following "binge-

like" alcohol exposure during the neonatal brain growth spurt. *Neurotoxicol Teratol., 13*:69–74.

[22] Miller M, Potempa G. (1990). Numbers of neurons and glia in mature rat somatosensory cortex: effects of prenatal exposure to ethanol. *J Comp Neurol.*, 293:92–102.

[23] West J, Dewey S, Pierce D, Black A Jr. (1984). Prenatal and early postnatal exposure to ethanol permanently alters the rat hippocampus. *Ciba Found Symp.*, 105:8–25.

[24] Boyadjieva N, Sarkar D. (2010). Role of microglia in ethanol's apoptotic action on hypothalamic neuronal cells in primary cultures. *Alcohol Clin Exp Res.*, 34:1835–1842.

[25] Guizzetti M, Zhang X, Goeke C, Gavin D. (2015). Corrigendum: "glia and neurodevelopment: focus on fetal alcohol spectrum disorders" *Front Pediatr.*, 3:27.

[26] Merighi S, Gessi S, Varani K, Fazzi D, Mirandola P, Borea P. (2012). Cannabinoid CB(2) receptor attenuates morphine-induced inflammatory responses in activated microglial cells. *Br J Pharmacol.,* 166:2371–2385.

[27] Chen C, Kuhn P, Advis J, Sarkar D. (2006). Prenatal ethanol exposure alters the expression of period genes governing the circadian function of beta-endorphin neurons in the hypothalamus. *J Neurochem.*, 97, 1026–1033.

[28] Baker R, Shoemaker W. (1995). Effect of prenatal ethanol and stress on levels of beta-endorphin in different brain regions of the rat. *Alcohol Clin Exp Res.,* 19:727–734.

[29] Sarkar D, Kuhn P, Marano J, Chen C, Boyadjieva N. (2007). Alcohol exposure during the developmental period induces beta-endorphin neuronal death and causes alteration in the opioid control of stress axis function. *Endocrinology,* 148:2828–2834.

[30] Scott H, Zoeller R, Rudeen P. (1995). Acute prenatal ethanol exposure and luteinizing hormone-releasing hormone messenger RNA expression in the fetal mouse brain. *Alcohol Clin Exp Res.*, 19:153–159.

[31] Lee S, Schmidt D, Tilders F, Rivier C. (2000). Increased activity of the hypothalamic-pituitary-adrenal axis of rats exposed to alcohol in utero: role of altered pituitary and hypothalamic function. *Mol Cell Neurosci.*, 16:515–528.

[32] Barson J, Morganstern I, Leibowitz S. (2010). Galanin and consummatory behavior: special relationship with dietary fat, alcohol and circulating lipids. *EXS.*, 102:87–111.

[33] Stettner G, Kubin L, Volgin D. (2011). Antagonism of orexin 1 receptors eliminates motor hyperactivity and improves homing response acquisition in juvenile rats exposed to alcohol during early postnatal period. *Behav Brain Res.*, 221:324–328.

[34] Rojas J, Vigueras R, Reyes G, Rojas P, Cintra L, Aguilar-Roblero R. (1999). Morphological changes produced by acute prenatal exposure to ethanol on the immunoreactive vasoactive intestinal polypeptide cells of the suprachiasmatic nucleus of the rat. *Proc West Pharmacol Soc.*, 42:75–76.

[35] Boyadjieva N, Sarkar D. (2010). Role of microglia in ethanol's apoptotic action on hypothalamic neuronal cells in primary cultures. *Alcohol Clin Exp Res.*, 34:1835–1842.

[36] Cohen-Kerem R, Koren G. (2003). Antioxidants and fetal protection against ethanol teratogenicity. I. Review of the experimental data and implications to humans. *Neurotoxicol Teratol.*, 25:1–9.

[37] Ramachandran V, Watts L, Maffi S, Chen J, Schenker S, Henderson G. (2003). Ethanol-induced oxidative stress precedes mitochondrially mediated apoptotic death of cultured fetal cortical neurons. *J Neurosci Res.*, 74:577–588.

[38] Reinke L, Lai E, DuBose C, McCay P. (1987). Reactive free radical generation *in vivo* in heart and liver of ethanol-fed rats: correlation with radical formation *in vitro*. *Proc Natl Acad Sci USA*, 84:9223–92227.

[39] Chao C, Hu S, Molitor T, Shaskan E, Peterson P. (1992). Activated microglia mediate neuronal cell injury via a nitric oxide mechanism. *J Immunol.*, 149:2736–2741.

[40] Colton C, Gilbert D. (1987). Production of superoxide anions by a CNS macrophage, the microglia. *FEBS Lett.*, 223:284–288.

[41] Min K, Jou I, Joe E. (2003). Plasminogen-induced IL-1beta and TNF-alpha production in microglia is regulated by reactive oxygen species. *Biochem Biophys Res Commun.*, 312:969–974.

[42] Wang H, Park U, Kim S, Lee J, Kim S, Gwag B, Lee Y. (2008). Free radical production in CA1 neurons induces MIP-1alpha expression, microglia recruitment, and delayed neuronal death after transient forebrain ischemia. *J Neurosci.*, 28:1721–1727.

[43] Boyadjieva N., Sarkar D. (2013). Microglia play a role in ethanol-induced oxidative stress and apoptosis in developing hypothalamic neurons. *Alcohol Clin Exp Res.*, 37 (2):252–262.

[44] Ramachandran V, Perez A, Chen J, Senthil D, Schenker S, Henderson GI. (2001). *In utero* ethanol exposure causes mitochondrial dysfunction, which can result in apoptotic cell death in fetal brain: a potential role for 4-hydroxynonenal. *Alcohol Clin Exp Res.*

[45] Dringen R, Kussmaul L, Gutterer J, Hirrlinger J, Hamprecht B. (1999). The glutathione system of peroxide detoxification is less efficient in neurons than in astroglial cells. *J Neurochem.*, 72:2523–2530.

[46] Wu D, Cederbaum A. (2001). Removal of glutathione produces apoptosis and necrosis in HepG2 cells overexpressing CYP2E1. *Alcohol Clin Exp Res.*, 25:619–628.

[47] Maffi S, Rathinam M, Cherian P, Pate W, Hamby-Mason R, Schenker S. Henderson G. (2008). Glutathione content as a potential mediator of the vulnerability of cultured fetal cortical neurons to ethanol-induced apoptosis. *J Neurosci Res.*, 86:1064–1076.

[48] Watts L, Rathinam M, Schenker S, Henderson G. (2005). Astrocytes protect neurons from ethanol-induced oxidative stress and apoptotic death. *J Neurosci Res.*, 80:655–666.

[49] Block M, Zecca L, Hong J. (2007). Microglia-mediated neurotoxicity: uncovering the molecular mechanisms. *Nat Rev Neurosci.*, 8:57–69.

[50] Streit W, Mrak R, Griffin W. (2004). Microglia and neuro-inflammation: a pathological perspective. *J Neuroinflammation*, 1:14.

[51] Combs C, Johnson D, Cannady S, Lehman T, Landreth G. (1999). Identification of microglial signal transduction pathways mediating a neurotoxic response to amyloidogenic fragments of betaamyloid and prion proteins. *J Neurosci.*, 19:928–939.

[52] McDonald D, Brunden K, Landreth G. (1997). Amyloid fibrils activate tyrosine kinase-dependent signaling and superoxide production in microglia. *J Neurosci.*, 17:2284–2294.

[53] Zou J, Crews F. (2010). Induction of innate immune gene expression cascades in brain slice cultures by ethanol: key role of NF-κB and proinflammatory cytokines. *Alcohol Clin Exp Res.*, 34:777– 789.

[54] Sarkar D, Kuhn P, Marano J, Chen C, Boyadjieva N. (2007). Alcohol exposure during the developmental period induces beta-endorphin neuronal death and causes alteration in the opioid control of stress axis function. *Endocrinology*, 148:2828–2834.

[55] Lee S, Schmidt D, Tilders F, Rivier C. (2000). Increased activity of the hypothalamic-pituitary-adrenal axis of rats exposed to alcohol in utero: role of altered pituitary and hypothalamic function. *Mol Cell Neurosci.*, 16:515–528.

[56] Zhang X, Sliwowska J, Weinberg J. (2005). Prenatal alcohol exposure and fetal programming: effects on neuroendocrine and immune function. *Exp Biol Med* (Maywood), 230:376–388.

[57] Logan R, Wynne O, Maglakelidze G, Zhang C, O'Connell S, Boyadjieva N, Sarkar D. (2015). β-Endorphin neuronal trans-plantation into the hypothalamus alters anxiety-like behaviors in prenatal alcohol-exposed rats and alcohol-non-preferring and alcohol-preferring rats. *Alcohol Clin Exp Res.*, 39(1):146–157.

[58] Boyadjieva N, Ortigüela M, Arjona A, Cheng X, Sarkar D. (2009). Beta-endorphin neuronal cell transplant reduces corticotropin releasing hormone hyperresponse to lipopolysaccharide and eliminates natural killer cell functional deficiencies in fetal alcohol exposed rats. *Alcohol Clin Exp Res.*, 33(5):931–937.

[59] Shrivastava P, Cabrera M., Chastain L, Boyadjieva N, Jabbar S, Franklin T, Sarkar D. (2017). Mu-opioid receptor and delta-opioid receptor differentially regulate microglial inflammatory response to control proopiomelanocortin neuronal apoptosis in the hypothalamus: effects of neonatal alcohol. *J Neuroinflammation*, 14: 83.

In: Fetal Alcohol Syndrome
Editor: Doug Knight

ISBN: 978-1-53614-602-8
© 2018 Nova Science Publishers, Inc.

Chapter 4

LONG-TERM EFFECTS OF FETAL ALCOHOL EXPOSURE ON THE IMMUNE SYSTEM

Nadka I. Boyadjieva[*], *MD, PhD, DSci,*
Miroslava G. Varadinova, MD, PhD
and Rositza D. Metodieva
Department of Pharmacology and Toxicology, Medical Faculty,
Medical University, Sofia, Bulgaria

ABSTRACT

Limited human studies have been conducted on the immune status of children with fetal alcohol spectrum disorder (FASD). The present review is aimed to fill up these gaps in knowledge. The chapter discusses various long-term effects of drinking during pregnancy on the immune and the neuroimmune systems of the developing fetus, baby and child. The results suggest that fetal alcohol exposure (FAE) induces long-term defects in the immunity and susceptibility to various infections. Mechanisms of impaired immune proliferation and function in FASD are a subject of the review. Chronic alcohol exposure in utero interferes with

---

[*] Corresponding Author Email: nadkaboyadjieva@gmail.com.

the normal T-cell and B-cell development of the fetus, which may increase the risk of infections during childhood and adult development. Influenza virus infection as well as increased risk for severe and fetal respiratory infections are illustrated in the long-term effects of FAE. Recognition of neuroimmunological dysfunctions due to developmental ethanol exposure and their lasting harmful effects in the early infancy and in the adulthood are also discussed in this chapter.

EFFECTS OF ALCOHOL EXPOSURE ON NK CELLS

Chronic alcohol intake affects NK cells in humans. Alcoholic patients with chronic active hepatitis and cirrhosis have low NK activity [1, 2]. Charpentier et al. (1984) found that NK cell activity was impaired only in alcoholic subjects with inactive cirrhosis [3]. It is unclear whether the immunological abnormalities in human alcoholics result from direct ethanol exposure or generalized malnutrition and toxicity of alcohol on the liver [4, 5, 6]. Saxena et al. (1980) observed enhanced NK cell activity in peripheral blood lymphocytes from alcoholic subjects despite various compounding factors such as malnutritional status, smoking, drug addiction, acute and chronic diseases, etc. [7]. Cirrhotic patients with severe malnutrition showed a decrease in NK cell activity. The combination of chronic alcohol intake and acute or chronic disease in patients plays a role in the function of NK cells. It is well known that alcohol abuse individuals may suffer from frequent viral infections which also affect the immune responses including NK cell function. In the opposite, chronic alcoholics who were well nourished and free of underlying diseases had no demonstrable abnormality in immune function, including NK cell activity [8]. Cook et al. (1997) showed a loss of NK cells in alcoholics with liver disease and low NK cell activity in alcoholics without liver disease [9].

A lot of data on the acute and chronic effects of ethanol on NK cells were obtained from animal studies. The relevance of rodent models of chronic alcohol intake to NK cells in humans exposed to alcohol is unknown. Assessments of NK cell activity in humans is complicated by the fact that many patients use various drugs or tobacco that are known to affect NK cell activity [10, 11]. For example, NK cell activity was decreased in depressed patients with alcoholism and treated with antidepressants [12]. However, different animal models of alcohol abuse were developed to demonstrate various harmful effects of alcohol including its effects on the immune system. In a binge drinking animal model Wu and Pruett (1994; 1996) showed an inhibition of the NK cell cytolytic activity and a decrease in the cell percentage and number in mice [13, 14]. According to various studies in which the nutritional status and the amount of ethanol intake were calculated, mice treated with high doses of ethanol (20% in the drinking water) showed inhibition of the NK cell cytolytic activity [15, 16, 17].

The role of β-endorphin (β-EP) in ethanol-altered NK cell cytolytic activity was published. Rats treated with ethanol for 1 wk showed an increase in hypothalamic and plasma levels of immunoreactive (IR)-β-EP, but displayed no significant effect on NK cell activity, as compared with those in pair-fed and ad libitum-fed animals [18]. Animals treated with ethanol for 2, 3, or 4 wk showed decreased hypothalamic and plasma levels of IR-β-EP and decreased splenic NK cell activity. In vitro exposure of splenic lymphocytes obtained from control animals to various concentrations of β-EP increased NK cell activity. Results from various studies on effects of ethanol on hypothalamic β-EP are in agreement with studies on rats [19, 20, 21, 22]. Acute treatment with ethanol stimulated hypothalamic content of β-EP and its precursor proopiomelanocortin (POMC) mRNA, whereas chronic treatment with ethanol reduced β-EP and POMC mRNA levels in this tissue. Similar biphasic actions of ethanol on β-EP and POMC mRNA levels were observed in hypothalamic cells in primary cultures [23, 24, 25, 26]. Additionally, the role of β-EP in ethanol-modulated NK cell function was evaluated in vivo by determining the effects of a hypothalamic administration of β-EP or naltrexone on splenic NK cell activity. It is well known that a large number of β-EP terminals and β-EP-sensitive receptors are localized in the paraventricular nucleus (PVN) of the hypothalamus [27, 28, 29, 30]. In our previous studies, opioid peptide and its blocker were infused into the PVN of alcohol-treated and non-alcohol-treated rats and the NK cytolytic activity was measured. Our results demonstrated that the β-EP infusion into the PVN increased the NK cell cytolytic activity in ad libitum- or pair-fed control animals. The infusion of the opioid peptide into the PVN failed to increase the NK cell activity in animals fed with an alcohol diet for a period of 2 weeks. PVN administration of the opiate blocker naltrexone in the control pair-fed animals significantly inhibited the NK cell activity, but did not affect the NK cell function in alcohol-fed animals.

Taken together, data obtained from in vivo studies suggest that chronic alcohol exposure of rats may decrease the plasma levels of β-EP as well as the activity of NK cells. The stimulatory action of β-EP on the NK cell function could occur by increasing their killing activity or by increasing their cytokine secretion. The role of the β-EP peptide in the immune system is illustrated also by its capacity to enhance the splenic lymphocyte proliferation in response to concanavalin A together with the increase of NK cell activity [31, 32, 33, 34]. It is known that IR-β-EP is present in lymphocytes [35] and in macrophages [36]. Additionally, the positive association between the changes of the NK cell function and the hypothalamic β-EP levels in ethanol-treated animals provides evidence for an involvement of the opioid peptide in the regulation of the NK cell function. This view is further supported by using opioid antagonists in both in vivo and in vitro studies. Results demonstrated that β-EP stimulated the NK cell function, which was blocked by the opiate antagonist naltrexone. The ability of morphine and enkephaline to affect various types of immune cells has been documented previously [37, 38, 39, 40, 41]. There is data that the lymphocytes possess ∂, κ, and μ opioid receptors [42]. It has been shown that endogenous opioids up-regulate human and rat NK cell activity via receptor mechanism of action [31, 32]. Additionally, POMC mRNA transcript has been identified in splenic lymphocytes [43, 44]. Both acetylated and nonacetylated β-EP are produced in splenic lymphocytes [36]. There is a difference between the effects of morphine and the enkephalines on the NK cells. Some studies demonstrated that treatment with morphine decreased NK cell activity [39, 40], whereas data from other studies supported the hypothesis that enkephalines increased the NK cell activity or had no effect [37, 38]. Thereafter, it is probably due to the role of various opioid receptors in the mechanisms of regulation of the NK cytolytic activity in the presence or not of alcohol.

It has also been shown that acute ethanol treatment elevates secretion of hormones like corticosterone and the hypothalamic corticotropin-releasing hormone [45, 46, 47]. Various studies in rats suggest that corticotropin-releasing hormone activates the sympathetic nervous system and releases norepinephrine to inhibit the NK cell function [48, 49, 50]. In contrast, the inhibitory effects of glucocorticoids on the NK cell function is not clear and remains to be evaluated in humans [51, 52, 53].

EFFECTS OF FETAL ALCOHOL EXPOSURE ON THE IMMUNE SYSTEM

Alcohol is one of the most common teratogenic agents. Alcohol crosses the placenta and can directly affect developing fetal cells and tissues. Consumption of alcohol during pregnancy has been widely associated with various adverse effects in the developing fetus, including premature birth, multiple birth defects, low birth weight, neuro-developmental disorders etc. It is well established that the exposure to alcohol during gestation can lead to a constellation of long lasting disabilities that include cognitive (i.e., intellectual ability, learning, and memory), behavioral (e.g., mood, attention, and impulse control) as well as immune dysfunctions. Recent studies suggest that the consumption of alcohol during pregnancy is causing lifelong effects on the neuroimmune functions. The most widely known consequences of prenatal alcohol exposure were clearly identified in neurobehavioral outcomes. Taken together, all diagnosed malformations and dysfunctions in babies born by mothers who have consumed alcohol during pregnancy were collectively named Fetal Alcohol Spectrum Disorder (FASD). There is a severe form of FASD, first described by Jones and Smith in 1973, named Fetal Alcohol Syndrome (FAS). FASD is characterized in various symptoms that not only capture FAS, but also alcohol-related neurodevelopmental disorder, and alcohol-related birth defects [54, 55]. Additionally, multiple clinical reports and case studies indicate that children with FASD frequently face secondary medical disabilities related to immune dysregulation (i.e., autoimmune or inflammatory reactivity, infections, etc.).

Alterations in the immune function may be one of the long-term consequences of fetal programming in alcohol consuming pregnant women [56]. Alcohol may have indirect effects on the immune system of fetuses through increased risk of premature birth, which itself is a risk factor for immune-related problems in babies and children. Human studies assessed that children diagnosed with FAS and neonates prenatally exposed to alcohol experienced a number of incidence of infection and immune-related pathologies, such as urinary tract infection, pneumonia, meningitis and the chronic autoimmune neuromuscular disease, myasthenia gravis [57, 58, 59]. Long-term effects of alcohol consumption on fetuses are expressed as peripheral immune system dysregulation in children [57, 60, 61]. McGill et al. (2009) published that fetal exposure to ethanol had long-term effects on the severity of influenza virus infections [62]. FASD has also been associated with increased severity in autoimmune arthritis and a susceptibility to developing a prostate cancer [63]. Additionally, various stages of dysregulation of cell-mediated immune responses have been reported with diminished T cell-proliferative responses [60, 64]. In a review of 13 documented cases of FASD, an increased incidence of life-threatening bacterial infections as well as a propensity to minor infections was observed. Maternal alcohol consumption increases circulating proinflammatory cytokine exposure to the fetus [58]. There is a hypothesis that alcohol levels persist longer in the fetal blood than in the maternal one (due to a not well-developed metabolism of the alcohol in the fetus) [59], and maybe the circulating fetal proinflammatory cytokines from alcohol exposure reprogram the inflammatory responses long after birth. An impairment of the immunity may explain the increased susceptibility to infections in FASD. Kim et al. (1999) demonstrated the effects of prenatal exposure to alcohol on the release of adrenocorticotropic hormone, corticosterone, and proinflammatory cytokines [61]. Based on current supporting evidence, various studies suggest that prenatal alcohol exposure is altering neurodevelopmental mechanisms of the toll-like receptor 4 (TLR4) on behavioral and cognitive dysfunctions associated with alcohol-induced neuroinflammatory damage [65]. Alcohol-induced TLR4-mediated signaling activates the NFκB pathway in microglia and astrocytes and leads to production of various inflammatory cytokines. Alcohol may alter neuroimmune responses followed by subsequent immune activation in fetuses via TLRs. Terasaki LS and Schwarz JM (2017) compared the impact of prenatal and subsequent adult alcohol exposure on pro-inflammatory cytokine expression in brain regions and documented the changes in the simple recognition memory [66]. The results demonstrated that a number of children with FASD had episodes of memory dysfunctions. Alcohol induced an increase in adhesion molecules such as vascular cell adhesion molecule-1 (VCAM-1). VCAM-1 binds to the very late antigen-4 (VLA-4) on leukocytes and the leukocyte function-associated antigen-1 (LFA-1) may facilitate and increase the magnitude of peripheral leukocyte migration across the brain blood barrier (BBB), following subsequent immune activation. This leads to neuroimmune consequences as well as to neuroinflammation. Prenatal alcohol exposure increases the C–C motif chemokine ligand-2 (CCL2) production in the CNS and CCL2 acts on peripheral leukocytes to recruit them to the CNS [67, 68, 69, 70]. Topper and Valenzuela (2014) demonstrated the effect of repeated alcohol exposure during the third trimester-equivalent on messenger RNA levels for interleukin-1 beta, CCL2, and interleukin 10 in the developing rat brain after injection of lipopolysaccharide [71]. Data from various studies suggest that a moderate prenatal alcohol exposure might be less disruptive to the neurodevelopment and to the neuroimmune system of FASD diagnosed children than binge-like exposures [71, 72, 73]. Additionally, our experimental studies demonstrated that pups of rats treated with alcohol during pregnancy had low cytolytic activity of NK cells of spleen and low concentration of INF in blood.

Alcohol crosses the placenta and can directly affect developing fetal cells and tissues. The most plausible hypothesis whereby alcohol decreases prenatal growth, is via hypoxia which interferes with cellular processes that require oxygen, such as placental transport and protein synthesis [74, 75]. There are two basic mechanisms in alcohol-induced fetal injury and somatic pathologies as following: (1) directly, via ethanol and/or acetaldehyde toxicity [76], and (2) indirectly, via ethanol-induced placental injury [77] and selective fetal malnutrition [78]. In vivo and in vitro experiments have demonstrated that transient ethanol exposure causes oxidative stress both in rat placenta [79, 80] and in human placental villous tissue [81]. Oxidative stress occurs when there is an imbalance between the production of reactive oxygen species (ROS) and the ability of the biological system to detoxify ROS [82, 83]. Oxidative stress is an essential part of the innate immune response to alcohol exposure in the developing CNS [84]. Fetal exposure to alcohol has been demonstrated to increase lipid peroxidation and oxidative stress markers like superoxide dismutase, catalase, reduced glutathione, and nitric oxide in the hippocampus and cerebral cortex of alcohol-treated rodents [85]. In addition, oxidative stress is accompanied by neurodegeneration and hence, alcohol-induced oxidative imbalances may contribute to the etiology of FASD. Alterations in the developing neuroimmune functions due to oxidative stress contribute to persistent neuropathological CNS dysfunction and are suggested as one of the long-term consequences of prenatal alcohol exposure. We have previously demonstrated that microglia may play an essential role in the ethanol-induced oxidative stress in developing neurons [86]. Normally, microglia are the primary immune cells in the CNS which maintain the homeostasis and have a neuroprotective role. However, when microglial cells are chronically activated they may be toxic to the neurons and contribute to the pathological mechanisms associated with neuro-inflammatory and neurodegenerative disorders. The dysfunctional neuroimmune response following fetal exposure to ethanol is suggested to have detrimental effects on the immature microglial populations in the developing brain, the lasting effects of which will increase the vulnerability of the adult brain to injury and infection.

Lots of evidence provided theories for the disruptive effects of alcohol on the developing neuroimmune system. Although the effects of fetal exposure to alcohol on the adult innate immune system are complex, taken together, these studies suggest that fetal alcohol exposure increases the vulnerability of adult peripheral and central immune mechanisms to injury and disease.

REFERENCES

[1] Vierling, J., Nelson, D., Strober W., Bundy, B. (1977). In vitro cell-mediated cytotoxicity in primary biliary cirrhosis and chronic hepatitis. *J. Clin. Invest.,* 60: 1116.

[2] Serdengecti, S., Jones, D., Holdstock, G., Wright, R. (1981). Natural killer activity in patients with biopsy-proven liver disease. *Clin. Exp. Immunol.,* 45: 361.

[3] Charpentier, B., Franco, D., Paci, L., Charra, M., Martin, B., Vuitton, D., Fries, D. (1984). Deficient natural killer cell activity in alcoholic cirrhosis. *Clin. Exp. Immunol.,* 58: 107.

[4] Shaw, S., Lieber, C. (1978). Plasma amino acid abnormalities in the alcoholic: respective role of alcohol, nutrition and liver injury. *Gastroenterology,* 74: 677.

[5] Yew, M., Moore, S., Biesele, M. (1981). Effects of chronic "moderate" alcohol consumption on vitamins A and C status of male Sprague-Dawley rats. *Nutr. Rep. Int.,* 23: 427.

[6] Neville, J., Eagles, J., Samson, G., Olson, R. (1968). Nutrition status of alcoholics. *Am. J. Clin. Nutr.,* 21:1329.

[7] Saxena, Q., Mezey, E., Adler, W. (1980). Regulation of natural killer activity in vivo: the effect of alcohol consumption on human peripheral blood natural killer activity. *Int. J. Cancer,* 26: 413.

[8] Kronfol, Z., Nair, M., Hill, E., Kroll, P., Brower, K., Greden, J. (1993). Immune function in alcoholism: a controlled study. *Alcoholism,* 17: 279.

[9] Cook, R., Li, F., Vandersteen, D., Ballas, Z., Cook, B., LaBrecque, D. (1997). Ethanol and natural killer cells: activity and immuno-phenotype in alcoholic humans. *Alcohol. Clin. Exp. Res.,* 21: 974.

[10] Ferson, M., Edwards, A., Lind, A., Milton, G., Hersey, P. (1979). Low natural killer-cell activity and immunoglobulin levels associated with smoking in human subjects. *Int. J. Cancer,* 23: 603.

[11] Klimas, N., Morgan, R., Blaney, N., Chitwood, D., Page, J., Milles, K., Fletcher, M. (1990). Alcohol and immune function in HIV-1 seronegative, HTLV- I/II seronegative and positive men on methadone. *Prog. Clin. Biol. Res.,* 325: 103.

[12] Irwin, M., Caldwell, C., Smith, T., Brown, S., Schuckit, M., Gillin, J. (1990). Major depressive disorder, alcoholism, and reduced natural killer cell cytotoxicity. *Arch. Gen. Psychiatry,* 47: 713.

[13] Wu, W., Pruett, S. (1994). Ethanol decreases the number and activity of splenic natural killer cells in a mouse model for binge drinking. *J. Pharmacol. Exp. Ther.,* 271: 722.

[14] Wu, W., Pruett, S. (1996). Suppression of splenic natural killer cell activity in a mouse model for binge drinking: role of the neuroendocrine system. *J. Pharmacol. Exp. Ther.,* 278: 1331.

[15] Blank, S., Duncan, D., Meadows, G. (1991). Suppression of natural killer cell activity by ethanol consumption and food restriction. *Alcohol. Clin. Exp. Res.,* 15: 16.

[16] Gallucci, R., Pfister, L., Meadows, G. (1994). Effects of ethanol consumption on enriched natural killer cells from C57BL/6 mice. *Alcohol. Clin. Exp. Res.* 18: 625.

[17] Abdallah, R., Starkey, J., Meadows, G. (1982). Ethanol and related dietary effects on mouse natural killer cell activity. *Immunology,* 50: 131.

[18] Boyadjieva, N., Dokur, M., Advis, J., Meadows, G. and Sarkar, D. (2001). Chronic ethanol Inhibits NK cell cytolytic activity: Role of opioid peptide β-Endorphin. *J Immunol,* 167 (X): 5645-5652.

[19] Froehlich, J. (1993). Interaction between alcohol and the endogenous opioid system. In: Zakhari SS, editor. *Alcohol and the endocrine system. No. 23 of National Institute of Alcohol Abuse and Alcoholism series.* Bethesda (MD): US Government Printing Office; 1993. p. 21-35.

[20] Gianoulakis, C. (1990). Characterization of the effects of acute ethanol administration on the release of β-endorphin peptides by the rat hypothalamus. *Eur. J. Pharmacol.,* 180: 21.

[21] Gianoulakis, C. (1996). Implications of endogenous opioids and dopamine in alcoholism: human and basic science studies. *Alcohol Alcohol.,* 31 *(Suppl. 1)*:33.

[22] Vescovi, P., Coiro, V., Volpi, R., Gianni, A., Passeri, M. (1992). Plasma β-endorphin but not met-enkephalin levels are abnormal in chronic alcoholics. *Alcohol Alcohol.,* 27: 471.

[23] Sarkar, D., Minami, S. (1990). Effect of acute ethanol on β-endorphin secretion from rat fetal hypothalamic neurons in cultures. *Life Sci.,* 47: 31-36.

[24] Boyadjieva, N., Sarkar, D. (1994). Effects of chronic ethanol on β-endorphin secretion from hypothalamic neurons in primary cultures: evidence for ethanol tolerance, withdrawal and sensitization responses. *Alcohol. Clin. Exp. Res.,* 18: 1497.

[25] Reddy, B., Boyadjieva, N., Sarkar, D. (1995). Effect of ethanol, propanol, butanol and catalase enzyme blockers on β-endorphin secretion from primary cultures of hypothalamic neurons: evidence for mediatory role of acetaldehyde in ethanol stimulation of β-endorphin release. *Alcohol. Clin. Exp. Res.,* 19:339.

[26] Pastorcic, M., Boyadjieva, N., Sarkar, D. (1994). Comparison of the effects of ethanol and acetaldehyde on proopiomelanocortin mRNA expression and β-endorphin secretion from hypothalamic neurons in primary cultures. *Cell. Mol. Neurosci.,* 5: 580.

[27] Rossier, J., Vargo, T., Minick, S., Ling, N., Bloom, F., Guillemin, R. (1977). Regional dissociation of β-endorphin and enkephalin contents in rat brain and pituitary. *Proc. Natl. Acad. Sci., USA* 11: 5162.

[28] Mezey, E., Kiss, J., O'Donohue, T., Eskay, R., Palkovits M. (1988). Distribution of pro-opiomelanocortin derived peptides (ACTH, α-MSH, β-endorphin) in the rat hypothalamus. *Brain Res.,* 328: 341.

[29] Wilcox, J., Roberts, J., Chronwall, B., Bishop, J., O'Donohue, T. 1986. Localization of proopiomelanocortin mRNA in functional

subsets of neurons defined by their axonal projections. *J. Neurosci. Res.,* 16: 89.

[30] O'Donohue, T., Dorsa, D. (1982). The opiomelanotropinergic neuronal and endocrine systems. *Peptides,* 3: 353.

[31] Kay, N., Allen, J., Morley, J. (1984). Endorphins stimulate normal human peripheral blood lymphocyte natural killer activity. *Life Sci.,* 35: 53.

[32] Mathews, P., Froelich, C., Sibbit, W., Jr, Bankhurst, A. (1983). Enhancement of natural cytotoxicity by β-endorphin. *J. Immunol.,* 130: 1658.

[33] Mandler, R., Biddison, W., Mandler, R., Serrate, S. 1986. β-Endorphin augments the cytolytic activity and interferon production of NK cells. *J. Immunol.,* 136: 934.

[34] Froehlich, C., Bankhurst, A. (1984). The effect of β-endorphin on natural cytotoxicity and antibody-dependent cellular cytotoxicity. *Life Sci.,* 35: 261.

[35] Smith, E., Blalock, J. (1981). Human lymphocyte production of corticotropin and endorphin-like substances: association with leukocyte interferon. *Proc. Natl. Acad. Sci., USA* 78: 7530.

[36] Lolait, S., Clements, J., Markwick, A., Cheng, C., McNally, M., Smith, A., Funder, J. (1986). Pro-opiomelanocortin messenger ribonucleic acid and post-translational processing of β-endorphin in spleen macrophages. *J. Clin. Invest.,* 77: 1776.

[37] Oleson, D., Johnson, D. (1988). Regulation of human natural cytotoxicity by enkephalins and selective opiate agonists. *Brain Behav. Immun.,* 2: 171.

[38] Gabriovac, J., Antica, M., Osmak, M. (1992). In vivo bidirectional regulation of mouse natural killer (NK) cell cytotoxic activities by leu-enkephalins: reversibility by naloxone. *Life Sci.,* 50: 29.

[39] Shavit, Y., Lewis, J., Terman, G., Gale, R., Liebeskind, J. (1984). Opioid peptides mediate the suppressive effect of stress on natural killer cell cytotoxicity. *Science,* 223: 188.

[40] Freier, D., Fuchs, B. (1994). A mechanism of action for morphine-induced immunosuppression: corticosterone mediates morphine-

induced suppression of natural killer cell activity. *J. Pharmacol. Exp. Ther.,* 270: 1127.

[41] Weber, R., Pert, A. (1989). The periaqueductal gray matter mediates opiate-induced immunosuppression. *Science,* 245: 188.

[42] Hazum, E., Chang, K., Cuatrecases, P. (1979). Specific nonopiate receptors for β-endorphin. *Science,* 205:1033.

[43] Endo, Y., Sakato, T., Watanabe, S. (1985). Identification of proopiomelanocortin-producing cells in the rat pyloric antrum and duodenum by in situ mRNA-cDNA hybridization. *Biomed. Res.,* 6: 253.

[44] Westly, H., Kleiss, A., Kelly, K., Wong, P., Yuen, P. (1986). Newcastle disease virus-infected splenocytes express the proopio-melanocortin gene. *J. Exp. Med.,* 163: 1589.

[45] Rivier, C. (1995). Interaction between stress and immune signals on the hypothalamic-pituitary-adrenal axis of the rat: influence of drugs. D.K. Sarkar, Jr, and C.D. Barnes, Jr, eds. *The Reproductive Neuroendocrinology of Aging and Drug Abuse* 169 CRC Press, Boca Raton, FL.

[46] Rivier, C., Lee, S. (1996). Acute alcohol administration stimulates the activity of hypothalamic neurons that express corticotropin-releasing factor and vasopressin. *Brain Res.,* 726: 1.

[47] Rasmussen, D., Bryant, C., Boldt, B., Colasurdo, E., Levin, N., Wilkinson, C. (1998). Acute alcohol effects on opiomelano-cortinergic regulation. *Alcohol. Clin. Exp. Res.,* 22: 789.

[48] Irwin, M. (1994). Stress-induced immune suppression: role of brain corticotropin-releasing hormone and autonomic nervous system mechanisms. *Adv. Neuroimmunol.,* 4: 29.

[49] Irwin, M., Hauger, R., Brown, M. (1992). Central corticotropin-releasing hormone activates the sympathetic nervous system and reduces immune function: increased responsivity of the aged rat. *Endocrinology,* 131:1047.

[50] Nistico, G., Caroleo, M., Arbitrio, M., Pulvirenti, L. (1994). Corticotropin-releasing factor microinfused into locus coeruleus

produces electro-cortical desynchronization and mmunosuppression. *Neuroimmunomodulation,* 1: 135.

[51] Bodner, G., Ho A., Kreek, M. (1998). Effect of endogenous cortisol levels on natural killer cell activity in healthy humans. *Brain Behav. Immun.,* 12: 285.

[52] Gatti, G., Masera, R., Pallavicini, L., Sartori, M., Staurengi, A., Orlandi, F., Angeli, A. (1993). Interplay in vitro between ACTH, β-endorphin and glucocorticosteroids in the modulation of spontaneous and lymphokine-inducible human natural killer (NK) cell activity. *Brain Behav. Immun.,* 7: 16.

[53] Holbrook, N., Cox, W., Horner, H. (1983). Direct suppression of natural killer activity in human peripheral blood leukocyte cultures by glucocorticoids and its modulation by interferon. *Cancer Res.,* 43: 4019.

[54] Sokol, R., Delaney-Black V. and Nordstrom B. (2003). Fetal alcohol spectrum disorder. *JAMA,* 290: 2996–9.

[55] Bertrand, J., Floyd, L. and Weber, M. (2005). Fetal Alcohol Syndrome Prevention Team, Division of Birth Defects and Developmental Disabilities, National Center on Birth Defects and Developmental Disabilities, Disease Control and Prevention (CDC). Guidelines for identifying and referring persons with fetal alcohol syndrome. *MMWR Recomm Rep,* 54: 1–14.

[56] Mattson, S., Crocker, N. and Nguyen T. (2011). Fetal alcohol spectrum disorders: neuropsychological and behavioral features. *Neuropsychol Rev,* 21: 81–101.

[57] Chiappelli, F. and Taylor, A. (1995). The fetal alcohol syndrome and fetal alcohol effects on immune competence. *Alcohol,* 30: 259–62.

[58] Ahluwalia, B., Wesley, B., Adeyiga, O., Smith, M., Da-Silva, A. and Rajguru S. (2000). Alcohol modulates cytokine secretion and synthesis in human fetus: an in vivo and in vitro study. *Alcohol,* 21: 207–13.

[59] Burd, L., Blair, J. and Dropps, K. (2012). Prenatal alcohol exposure, blood alcohol concentrations and alcohol elimination rates for the mother, fetus and newborn. *J Perinatol,* 32: 652–9.

[60] Weinberg, J. and Jerrells, R. (1991). Suppression of immune responsiveness: sex differences in prenatal ethanol effects. *Alcohol Clin Exp Res,* 15: 525–31.

[61] Kim, C., Turnbull, A., Lee, S. and Rivier, C. (1999). Effects of prenatal exposure to alcohol on the release of adrenocorticotropic hormone, corticosterone, and proinflammatory cytokines. *Alcohol Clin Exp Res,* 23: 52–9.

[62] McGill, J., Meyerholz, D., Edsen-Moore, M., Young, B., Coleman, A., Schlueter, A., et al. (2009). Fetal exposure to ethanol has long-term effects on the severity of influenza virus infections. *J Immunol,* 182: 7803–8.

[63] Murugan, S., Zhang, C., Mojtahedzadeh, S. and Sarkar, D. (2013). Alcohol exposure in utero increases susceptibility to prostate tumorigenesis in rat offspring. *Alcohol Clin Exp Res,* 37: 1901–9.

[64] Zhang, X., Lan, N., Bach, P., Nordstokke, D., Yu, W., Ellis, L., et al. (2012). Prenatal alcohol exposure alters the course and severity of adjuvant-induced arthritis in female rats. *Brain Behav Immun,* 26: 439–50.

[65] Pascual, M., Balino, P., Alfonso-Loeches, S., Aragon, C. and Guerri, C. (2011). Impact of TLR4 on behavioral and cognitive dysfunctions associated with alcohol-induced neuroinflammatory damage. *Brain Behav Immun,* 25 (Suppl 1): 80–91.

[66] Terasaki, L. and Schwarz, J. (2017). Impact of prenatal and subsequent adult alcohol exposure on pro-inflammatory cytokine expression in brain regions necessary for simple recognition memory. *Brain Sci,* 7: 125.

[67] Lobo-Silva, D., Carriche, G., Castro, A., Roque, S. and Saraiva, M. (2016). Balancing the immune response in the brain: IL-10 and its regulation. *J Neuroinflammation,* 13: 297.

[68] Husemann, J., Loike, J., Anankov, R., Febbraio, M. and Silverstein, S. (2002). Scavenger receptors in neurobiology and neuropathology: their role on microglia and other cells of the nervous system. *Glia,* 40: 195–205.

[69] Carson, M., Doose, J., Melchior, B., Schmid, C. and Ploix, C. (2006). CNS immune privilege: hiding in plain sight. *Immunol Rev,* 213: 48–65.

[70] Sochocka, M., Diniz, B. and Leszek, J. (2017). Inflammatory response in the CNS: friend or foe? *Mol Neurobiol*, 54: 8071–89.

[71] Topper, L. and Valenzuela, C. (2014). Effect of repeated alcohol exposure during the third trimester-equivalent on messenger RNA levels for interleukin-1beta, chemokine (C-C motif) ligand 2, and interleukin 10 in the developing rat brain after injection of lipopolysaccharide. *Alcohol,* 48: 773–80.

[72] Falgreen Eriksen, H., Mortensen, E., Kilburn, T., Underbjerg, M., Bertrand, J. and Stovring, H., et al. (2012). The effects of low to moderate prenatal alcohol exposure in early pregnancy on IQ in 5-year-old children. *BJOG*, 119: 1191–200.

[73] Skogerbo, A., Kesmodel, U., Wimberley, T., Stovring, H., Bertrand, J., Landro, N., et al. (2012). The effects of low to moderate alcohol consumption and binge drinking in early pregnancy on executive function in 5-year-old children. *BJOG*, 119: 1201–10.

[74] Bosco, C., Diaz, E. (2012). Placental hypoxia and fetal development versus alcohol exposure in pregnancy. *Alcohol Alcohol*, 47: 109-117.

[75] Bosco, C. Alcohol and Xenobiotics in Placenta Damage. (2005). In Preedy, V. and Watson, R. (eds) *Comprehensive Handbook of Alcohol Related Pathology*. London: Elsevier Science, Vol. 2: 921-935.

[76] Henderson, G., Patwardhan, R., Hoyumpa, A. Jr, Schenker, S. (1981). Fetal alcohol syndrome: overview of pathogenesis. *Neurobehav Toxicol Teratol*, 3: 73-80.

[77] Clave, S., Joya, X., Salat-Batlle, J., Garcia-Algar, O., Vall, O. (2014). Ethanol cytotoxic effect on trophoblast cells. *Toxicol Lett*, 225: 216-221.

[78] Fisher, S., Karl, P. (1988). Maternal ethanol use and selective fetal malnutrition. *Recent Dev Alcohol,* 6: 277-289.

[79] Gundogan, F., Elwood, G., Longato, L., Tong, M., Feijoo, A., et al. (2008). Impaired placentation in fetal alcohol syndrome. *Placenta*, 29: 148-157.

[80] Gundogan, F., Elwood, G., Mark, P., Feijoo, A., Longato, L., et al. (2010). Ethanol-induced oxidative stress and mitochondrial dysfunction in rat placenta: relevance to pregnancy loss. *Alcohol Clin Exp Res*, 34: 415-423.

[81] Kay, H., Grindle, K., Magness, R. (2000). Ethanol exposure induces oxidative stress and impairs nitric oxide availability in the human placental villi: a possible mechanism of toxicity. *Am J Obstet Gynecol*, 182: 682-688.

[82] Rodrigo, R., Parra, M., Bosco, C., Fernández, V., Barja, P., et al. (2005). Pathophysiological basis for the prophylaxis of preeclampsia through early supplementation with antioxidant vitamins. *Pharmacol Ther*, 107: 177-197.

[83] Wells, P., McCallum, G., Chen, C., Henderson, J., Lee, C., et al. (2009). Oxidative stress in developmental origins of disease: teratogenesis, neurodevelopmental deficits, and cancer. *Toxicol Sci*, 108: 4-18.

[84] Kane, C., Phelan, K., Drew, P. (2012). Neuroimmune mechanisms in fetal alcohol spectrum disorder. *Dev Neurobiol*, 72:1302–1316.

[85] Tiwari, V., Chopra, K. (2011). Resveratrol prevents alcohol-induced cognitive deficits and brain damage by blocking inflammatory signaling and cell death cascade in neonatal rat brain. *J Neurochem*, 117:678–690.

[86] Boyadjieva, N., Sarkar, D. (2013). Microglia play a role in ethanol-induced oxidative stress and apoptosis in developing hypothalamic neurons. *Alcohol Clin Exp Res*. 37(2):252-262.

INDEX

methylation, ix, 20, 44, 45, 46, 47, 49, 50, 51, 53, 54, 55
mice, 34, 35, 36, 37, 39, 40, 42, 43, 45, 50, 53, 56, 75, 82
microRNA (miRNA, μRNA), ix, 20, 44, 45, 46, 48, 54, 56, 57
molecules, 44, 45, 60, 61, 62, 65, 79

N

nervous system, 5, 6, 9, 66, 87
neurodegeneration, 60, 61, 65, 66, 80
neurodegenerative disorders, 38, 80
neurodevelopmental disorders, 77
neuroimmune functions, 77, 80
neuronal cells, 46, 60, 62, 68, 69
neuronal plasticity, ix, 60
neuronal sensitivity, 64
neuron-microglia interactions, v, vii, ix, 59, 60, 61, 62
neurons, vii, ix, 46, 59, 60, 61, 62, 63, 64, 65, 67, 68, 70, 80, 83, 84, 85, 89
neuropathic pain, 67
nitric oxide, ix, 60, 64, 69, 80, 89
nitric oxide synthase, ix, 60
NK cells, 74, 76, 79, 84
noradrenergic system, 61, 66
normal pressure hydrocephalus, 53
nutritional status, 34, 75

O

oxidative damage, 38
oxidative stress, 38, 48, 63, 64, 69, 70, 80, 89

P

peripheral blood, 74, 81, 84, 86
peripheral nervous system, 60

phenotype, 13, 46, 60, 66
phosphatidylethanol (PEth), ix, 20, 24, 47, 52, 57
placenta, 30, 39, 77, 79, 89
placental growth factor (PLGF), 39, 47, 53
pregnancy, vii, viii, ix, x, 1, 3, 4, 6, 7, 8, 14, 16, 17, 20, 21, 23, 24, 25, 28, 30, 31, 32, 33, 34, 36, 37, 39, 40, 50, 51, 52, 53, 54, 57, 59, 73, 77, 79, 88, 89
preschool, vii, viii, 20, 21
prevention, 8, 15, 16, 17, 50, 64
pro-inflammatory, 62, 65, 79, 87

R

reactive oxygen, 63, 64, 70, 80
receptors, 37, 41, 61, 65, 67, 69, 75, 76, 85, 87
response, 22, 37, 40, 60, 61, 69, 71, 72, 76, 80, 88

S

secretion, 41, 65, 76, 77, 83, 86
sensitivity, 22, 27, 28, 31, 32, 33, 34, 39, 50, 51
serum, 22, 23, 26, 37, 39, 40, 43, 48, 49, 50, 53, 54
sex differences, 87
stress, 37, 39, 40, 48, 56, 61, 63, 64, 65, 68, 71, 80, 84, 85, 89
substance abuse, 11
suppression, 45, 85, 86
suprachiasmatic nucleus, 62, 69
susceptibility, viii, x, 57, 73, 78, 87
sympathetic nervous system, 77, 85
synaptic plasticity, 50, 60
syndrome, v, vii, viii, 1, 2, 6, 8, 9, 12, 13, 14, 15, 16, 17, 19, 20, 21, 41, 50, 56, 57, 77, 86, 88, 89